Habiba Debbabi
Mohamed Ben zayed

Quick sequential organ failure assessment in cirrhosis

Habiba Debbabi
Mohamed Ben zayed

Quick sequential organ failure assessment in cirrhosis

Interest of the score in infected cirrhotics

ScienciaScripts

Imprint

Cover image: www.ingimage.com

This book is a translation from the original published under ISBN 978-620-6-72836-8.

Publisher:
Sciencia Scripts
is a trademark of
Dodo Books Indian Ocean Ltd. and OmniScriptum S.R.L publishing group

120 High Road, East Finchley, London, N2 9ED, United Kingdom
Str. Armeneasca 28/1, office 1, Chisinau MD-2012, Republic of Moldova, Europe
Managing Directors: Ieva Konstantinova, Victoria Ursu
info@omniscriptum.com

Printed at: see last page
ISBN: 978-620-8-51089-3

Contents

1 INTRODUCTION

Cirrhosis is the consequence of all chronic liver disease. It is a frequent pathology and remains a major public health problem worldwide, due to its progressive course, which is grafted by the occurrence of frequent complications that can potentially jeopardise the vital prognosis. Infections, particularly bacterial infections, are one example, and are a frequent reason for admission of cirrhotic patients [1]. They are associated with an increased risk of progression to acute decompensation and multi-visceral failure, and expose cirrhotic patients to an increased risk of mortality [2]. This finding may explain the prolongation over time of hospital stays and costs incurred by this disease worldwide [3]. With a view to improving the management and prognosis of cirrhotic patients, several cirrhosis-specific severity scores have been used to identify these patients early and ensure effective management. The modified ChildPugh and MELD (Model for End-Stage Liver Disease) scores [4,5] have been the most widely used, but remain less effective in terms of assessing patient prognosis [5]. In this context, the SOFA (Sequential Organ Failure Assessment) score and its version adapted for patients with liver disease: the CLIF- SOFA [6] were validated at a consensus conference. These scores make it possible assess patient severity, predict prognosis and estimate the risk of in-hospital mortality according to initial severity. However, the complexity of the SOFA score and the need for biological samples limit its application outside intensive care units, leading to the development of a simplified version: the Quick SOFA (qSOFA) [7]. It consists of three variables (altered consciousness, systolic blood pressure (SBP) <100 mmHg and respiratory rate (RR) >22/min), each scored by one point and easily measured, particularly in emergency departments. The qSOFA is not a diagnostic criterion for sepsis, but a tool for rapid identification of the most serious patients or those likely to deteriorate. The combination of two out of three variables has demonstrated a predictive value in terms of mortality similar to that of the SOFA score [7].

The aim of our study was to assess the relevance of the qSOFA prognostic score, established on admission, in predicting mortality in cirrhotic patients with bacterial infection.

2 METHODS

1. Type of study

This is a retrospective, monocentric, descriptive study carried out between January 2016 and December 2020, i.e. over a period of 5 years, including all cirrhotic patients hospitalised in the Gastroenterology-Hepatology B department of La Rabta Hospital for an episode of bacterial infection.

2. Study population

2.1. Inclusion criteria :

All cirrhotic patients admitted to the Gastroenterology-Hepatology B department of La Rabta Hospital with a bacterial infection during the study period.

The diagnosis of cirrhosis was made on the basis of combination of clinical, biological, morphological (imaging or pulse elastometry) and endoscopic evidence, together with signs of hepatocellular insufficiency and portal hypertension.

2.2. Non-inclusion criteria

All cirrhotic patients with a history of progressive neoplastic pathology other than hepatocellular carcinoma (HCC) and/or had presented, at inclusion, an episode of upper GI haemorrhage (HDH), hepatorenal syndrome (HRS) and/or HCC. The diagnosis of SHR was retained according to the diagnostic criteria of the "European Association for the Study of the Liver" (EASL) published in 2018 [8](Appendix 1).

2.3. Exclusion criteria

The study did not include :

Patients whose files are incomplete and those lost to follow-up.

-Patients with a second episode bacterial infection or one of the following complications during the study period:

- An HDH
- An SHR
- HCC.

3. Data collection

For each patient included in the study, we recorded demographic, clinical, microbiological and paraclinical data, and calculated the qSOFA score retrospectively for each subject on the basis of clinical parameters collected on admission. Patients were followed for 12 months. Data were collected from the medical records and compiled on using a data collection form (Appendix 2). For all patients, the following data were collected:

3.1. Socio-demographic and anamnestic data :

+- Age

+ Type

+ Habits (smoking, alcohol or drug abuse)

+ Personal medical history (diabetes, hypertension, dyslipidaemia, coronary insufficiency, heart failure, respiratory insufficiency) and surgical history.

4- Data relating to cirrhosis (year of discovery, etiology of cirrhosis, mode of decompensation of cirrhosis on admission, Child Pugh score, MELD score)

+- Data relating to the first episode of infection: site of infection, results of microbiological samples,

antibiotic treatment, complications, length of hospital stay and in-hospital mortality at 6 and 12 months after the infectious episode.

The history included details of the various functional signs and the following reasons for consultation: fever, chills, asthenia, abdominal pain, diarrhoea, vomiting, dyspnoea, productive cough and urinary signs, as well as the length of time between the consultation and the onset of symptoms.

3.2. Clinical data :

The following clinical signs were investigated following the infectious episode: fever, general condition according to the WHO scale (Appendix 3), haemodynamic status (blood pressure and pulse), RF, jaundice, ascites, lower limb edema (LLE), neurological status with Glasgow Coma Score (GCS) (Appendix 4) and the possible presence of hepatic encephalopathy (HE).

3.3. Biological data :

We noted the various results of the biological tests requested on admission:

+- Blood count (CBC) with haemoglobin (Hb) (in g/dl), haematocrit (in %) and platelets (number/mm3).

An Hb level of <12 in women and <13 in men defines anaemia.

+- Haemostasis work-up with prothrombin rate (PT) and INR (International Normalized Ratio) and activated partial thromboplastin rate (APTT).

+ Liver function tests: aspartate aminotransferase (ASAT) in IU/L, alanine aminotransferase (ALAT) in IU/L, gamma-glutamyltransferase (GGT) in IU/L, alkaline phosphatase (PAL) in IU/L, total and conjugated bilirubin in mg/dl.

+- Albumin levels in g/L.
+- Kidney function: urea in mmol and creatinine in pmol/L.
+- Blood ionogram: natraemia and kalaemia in mmol/L.
Hyponatremia is considered to be present if the natraemia value was <130 mmol/L.
+ C-reactive protein (CRP) in mg/L.
We used a threshold of >10 to define an elevated CRP.

3.4. Data relating to the infectious episode :

3.4.1. Sites of infection :

- Urinary tract infection

- A urinary tract infection (UTI) was suspected in the presence of :
Evocative clinical signs (fever and/or urinary signs) or isolation of germs at a pathological threshold on urine cytobacteriological examination (UCO).
- Significant leucocyturia on ECBU (>10^4/ml)

- **Infection of ascites fluid**

Ascites fluid infection (EFI) was confirmed by cytobacteriological examination of the ascites fluid, taken during exploratory puncture of the ascites fluid (PELA), by a neutrophil count (PNN) > 250/mm3 in the ascites fluid.

- **Bronchopulmonary infection**

Acute pneumopathy was suspected in the presence of a combination of :
- Clinical criteria (fever > 37.8°C, tachycardia > 100 beats per minute, polypnoea > 25 cycles/minute, chest pain and absence of upper airway infection)
- Focal condensation on chest X-ray.

The diagnosis of acute bronchitis was based on the combination of fever, bronchial syndrome and the absence of condensation on chest X-ray.

- Other infections

Skin, osteoarticular, genital and ENT infections were selected on the basis of clinical, biological, microbiological and morphological criteria.

3.4.2. Sensitivity of the germs involved :

Bacteria are classified according to their sensitivity to different classes of antibiotics:

- Multi-sensitive bacteria (MSS): bacteria sensitive to several families of antibiotics (have acquired little or no resistance).
- Multi-resistant bacteria (MRB): bacteria that have accumulated acquired resistance to several families of antibiotics (> 3 different families, including beta-lactams).

3.4.3. Effectiveness of antibiotic therapy :

Response to antibiotic treatment was judged by improvement in clinical, biological, microbiological and radiological parameters. Clinical and biological parameters were assessed 48-72 hours after the initial antibiotic treatment. Clinical parameters were improvement in symptoms (apyrexia, improvement in haemodynamic status, improvement neurological disorders, etc.). Biological parameters were a reduction in inflammatory (WBC, PNN, CRP, etc.). Radiological parameters improvement radiological images if present.

3.4.4. Complications :

- **Septic shock :**

Shock is defined as persistent hypotension requiring vasopressors to maintain a mean arterial pressure > 65 mmHg, and a serum lactate level > 18 mg/dL [2 mmol/L], despite adequate volume resuscitation [9]. It is said to be septic when its origin is infectious.

- **Acute on Chronic Liver Failure:**

Acute on Chronic Liver Failure (ACLF) is defined by the combination of three elements: acute decompensation cirrhosis, one or more organ failures and a high mortality rate [8].

3.5. qSOFA score (Appendix 5) :

The qSOFA score has been proposed to identify the presence of organ failure in patients with suspected infection [9]. It comprises three clinical variables:

- Respiratory rate (RR) > 22
- Impairment of higher functions (confusion, disorientation), i.e. Glasgow Sign Score (GCS) <15
- Blood pressure (SAP) < 100 mmHg

One point is awarded for each of the preceding criteria, where present. This score is noted from 0 to 3. A number of points greater than or equal to two (> 2) defines a positive score. The score is said to be negative if it is less than two points (<2). A positive qSOFA identifies a patient at high risk mortality from sepsis [9]. For each patient in the study, the qSOFA score on admission was calculated retrospectively.

3.6 Evolution :

After the infectious episode, we assessed patient's progress. A favourable outcome was considered when :

- The disappearance of the infectious syndrome
- Cleaning X-ray images
- Negativation of a previously positive bacteriological sample.

- The absence of complications.

Progression is said to be unfavourable in cases of :

-Complications: septic shock, EH, onset or worsening of renal failure, ACLF, respiratory distress, etc.

-Deaths: mortality was assessed within the hospital and over a follow-up period of 6 to 12 months following the infectious episode. Overall mortality was defined as cumulative mortality over a 12-month follow-up period.

4. Statistical study :

The data were entered and analysed using SPSS software® for Windows version 20. We conducted :

4.1. Descriptive study :

We have calculated the :

- Qualitative variables: simple frequencies and relative frequencies (percentages)
- Quantitative variables: means, medians, standard deviations and distribution (extreme values: minimum and maximum).

4.2. Analytical study :

Comparisons were made using Student's t-test for quantitative variables and Pearson's chi-square test and Fisher's exact test for qualitative variables. We performed a univariate analysis using a logistic regression model including variables with a p-value of less than 0.2 in the univariate analysis. In all statistical tests, the significance level was set at 0.05.

The performance of the qSOFA score in terms of mortality by studying sensitivity and specificity using ROC curves and determining areas under the curves (AUROC).

5. Ethical considerations :

As our study was retrospective, consent was signed. But the confidentiality of medical data was respected. We have conflict of interest.

6. Bibliographic research :

A bibliographic search was carried out on the Pubmed and Science Direct websites using the following key words: cirrhosis, infection, qSOFA score, antibiotic therapy.

7. Ethical considerations

Strict anonymity of individual data was maintained throughout the study. The data was pseudonymised and only the principal investigator knew the identity of the patients. Given the retrospective nature of the study, it was not possible to obtain informed consent from patients.

There were no conflicts of interest in this work.

3 RESULTS

1. Descriptive study

1.1. Epidemiological characteristics of patients :

During the study period (January 2016 to December 2020), we hospitalised 145 cirrhotic patients with bacterial infections in the Gastro-Entero-Hepatology B department of the Rabta University Hospital.

Thirty-seven patients were not included in this study. These patients had a history of progressive neoplastic pathology other than HCC (n=6) and/or had, at inclusion, an episode of HDH (n=11), SHR (n=12) and/or HCC (n=8).

Forty-seven patients were excluded from the study. Excluded patients were those who developed a second episode of bacterial infection (n=15) or one of the following complications during the study period:

- One HDH (n=8).
- One SHR (n=7).
- One HCC (n=3).

Lost to follow-up (n=6) and incomplete files (n=8) were also excluded.

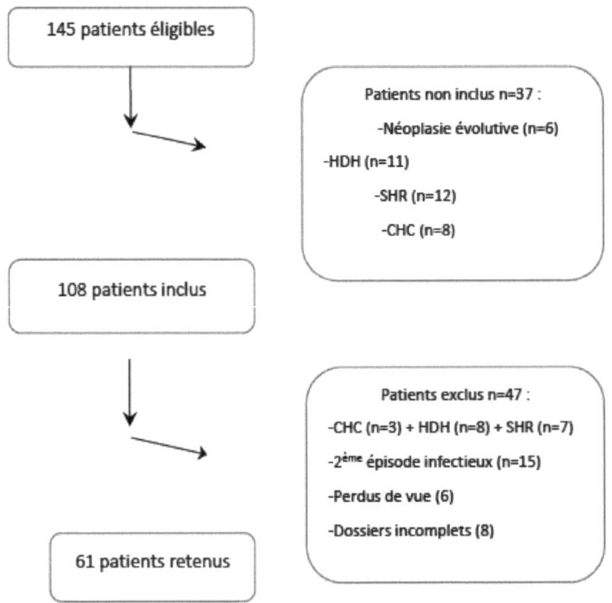

145 eligible patients

Patients not included n=37 :

-Progressive neoplasia (n=6)

-HDH (n=11)

-SHR (n=12) -CHC (n=8)

108 patients included

Patients excluded n=47 :

- HCC (n=3) + HDH (n=8) + SHR (n=7)
- 2th infectious episode (n=15)
- Lost and Found (6)
- Incomplete files (8)

61 patients selected

Figure 1: *Inclusion and exclusion criteria for the study population*

1.1.1.Age :

The mean age was 63±12 years [extremes: 25-85 years]. Forty-two patients (68.8%) were over 60 years of age. Figure 2 shows the distribution of patients by age group.

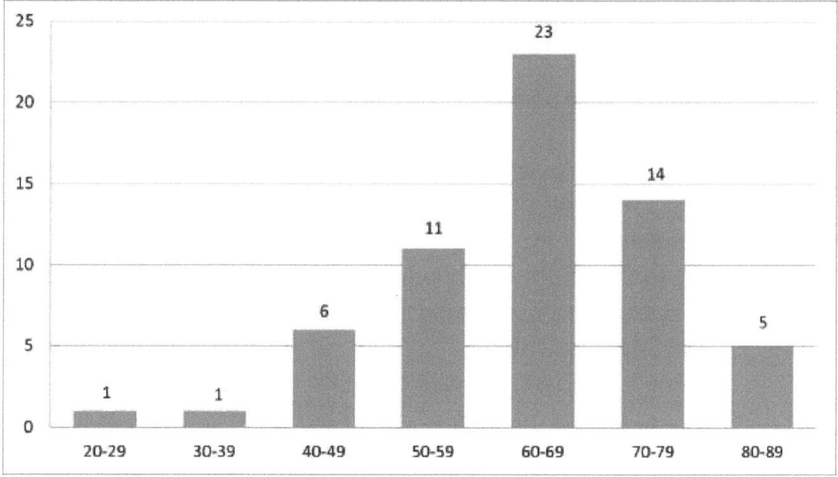

Figure 2: *Breakdown of patients by age group.*

1.1.2.Genre :

The patients were divided into 37 women (61%) and 24 men (39%), giving a gender ratio of 0.65 men to women. **(Figure 3).**

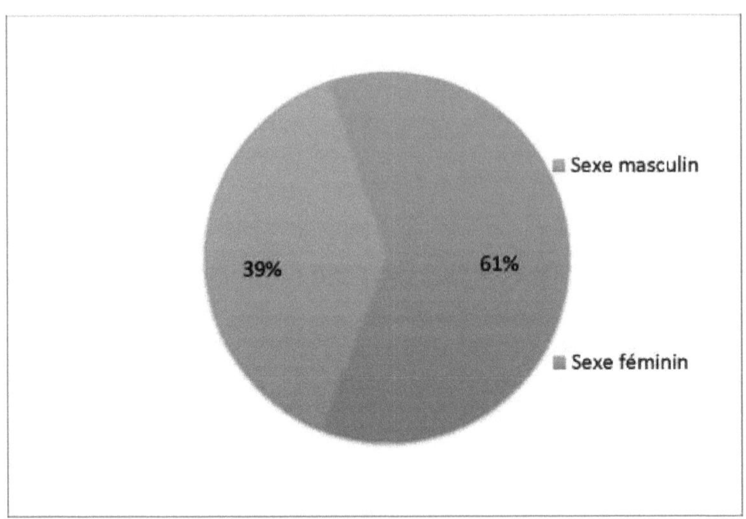

Figure 3: *Distribution of patients by gender.*

1.1.3. Habits :

Sixteen of our patients were smokers (26.2%). Chronic alcoholism exceeding 20 grams of alcohol per day, was noted in 2 patients (3.3%).

1.1.4. Comorbidities :

Thirty-seven patients had comorbidities (60.7%). The most frequent pathologies diabetes and hypertension, found respectively in 20 (32.8%) and 16 (26.2%) patients (Table I).

Table I. Main extra-hepatic medical co-morbidities

Associated pathologies	Number of cases	Percentage(%)
Diabetes	20	32,8
HTA	16	26,2
Non-ischaemic heart disease	5	8,2
Hypothyroi'die	4	6,6
Coronary insufficiency	4	6,6
Respiratory failure chronicle	4	6,6
Renal insufficiency chronicle	2	3,3
Lupus erythematosus systemic	2	3,3
Crohn's disease	1	1,6
Celiac disease	1	1,6

1.2 Clinical and biological data at the time of the episode

bacterial infection :

1.2.1. Circumstances of discovery :

The main signs of discovery of the infectious episode were ascitic or oedemato-ascitic decompensation (86.9%), abdominal pain (63.9%), asthenia (62.3%) and fever (52.5%) (Table II).

Table II. *Main circumstances in which bacterial infection is discovered*

Designs	Patients (n=61)	Percentage (%)
Ascitic decompensation or oedemato-ascitic	53	86,9
Abdominal pain	39	63,9
Asthenia	38	62,3
Fever	32	52,5
Urinary signs	24	39,3
EH	15	24,6
Dyspnoea	13	21,3
Cough	12	19,7
Vomiting	7	11,5
Chills	7	11,5
Diarrhoea	6	9,8
Inflammatory plaque of the lower limbs	3	4,9
Joint pain	2	3,3

*Several symptoms may be associated, and the total number of symptoms may vary.

patients can be more than 100%.

Consultation times ranged from 2 days to 150 days, with a median of 8 days [5-14].

1.2.2. Clinical examination :

General condition, assessed according to the WHO score, was 2 in 27 patients (44.3%). Twenty-three patients (37.7%) had a WHO score between 3 and 4, defining an altered general condition. Eleven cirrhotics had a WHO score between 0 and 1 (18%).

Consciousness was assessed using the Glasgow Coma Scale (GCS). This score was 15 in 53 patients (86.9%), 14 in 4 patients (6.6%), 12 in 3 patients (4.9%) and 11 in one patient (1.6%).

EH was found in 24 patients (39.3%). It was classified as grade 1 in 11 patients (18%), grade 2 in 9 patients (14.8%) and grade 3 in 4 patients

(6.6%).

Medium to large ascites was observed in 53 patients (86.9%), associated with renal IMO in 48 patients (78.8%). Nine patients (14.8%) had refractory ascites. Clinical examination data are summarised in Table III.

Table III. *Clinical examination data*

Clinical signs	Number (n=61)	Percentage (%)
Ascites	53	89,9
IMO	48	78,8
Low blood pressure	34	55,7
Polypnoea	29	47,5
EH	24	39,3
General state of health	23	37,7
Fever	22	36,1
Jaundice	13	21,3
Pleuresis	7	11,5
Bronchial rales	6	9,8
Signs of dehydration	5	8,2
Erysipelas	4	6,6
Erythematopultaceous throat	1	1,6
Leucorrhoea	1	1,6

1.2.3. Biological data :

Anaemia was the most frequent biological abnormality, found in 51 patients (83.7%).

Hyperleukocytosis was observed in 15 patients (24.6%).

CRP was elevated in 49 patients, or 80.3% of the study population. The mean level was 37.78 mg/L ± 32.56 (2-178 mg/L) and the median level was 30.6 mg/L [15-51.05].

IR (other than hepato-renal syndrome) was noted in 6 patients on admission (9.8%).

Hyponatremia was observed in 10 patients (16.4%).

Table IV. *Principal biological abnormalities*

Biological abnormality	Workforce	Percentage (%)
Anemia	51	83,7
Elevated CRP	49	80,3
Hyperleukocytosis	15	24,6
Hyponatremia	10	16,4
IR	6	9,8

1.3. Characteristics of cirrhotic disease :

1.3.1. Duration of cirrhosis at the time of infection bacterial :

The median time between the positive diagnosis of cirrhosis and the infectious episode was 24 months [11.5 - 45], with extremes ranging from 0 months to 300 months.

Infection was inaugural in 15% of cases (9 patients).

1.3.2. Etiology of cirrhosis :

The aetiologies cirrhosis were dominated by viral infections (63.9%), with a predominance of viral hepatitis C (HCV) (37.7%) and hepatitis B (HBV) (26.2%) (16 patients, including one B-D co-infection).

Autoimmune hepatitis (AIH) was observed in 7 patients (11.5%), including an overlapping syndrome of autoimmune hepatitis and primary biliary cholangitis (AIH-PBC).

Alcoholic cirrhosis was noted in two patients (3.3%).

The different aetiologies are summarised in the figure below (Figure 4).

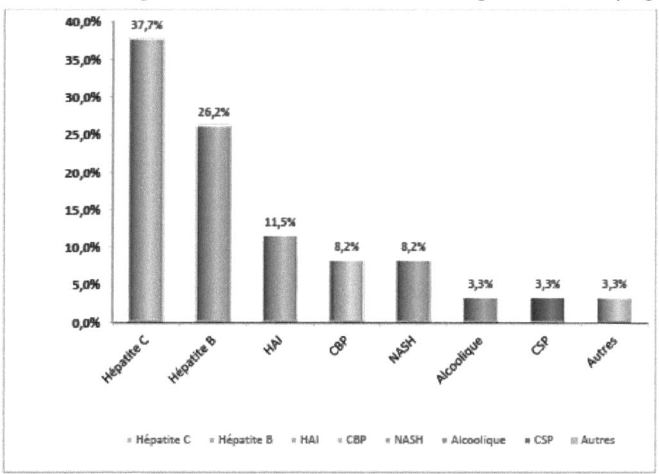

Figure 4: *Causes of cirrhosis.*

1.3.3. Severity of cirrhosis at the time of bacterial infection :

1.3.3.1. <u>Child Pugh score</u>

Thirty-one patients were classified asChild Pugh C (50.8%) and 23 patients (37.7%) Child Pugh B at the time of bacterial infection (Figure 5).

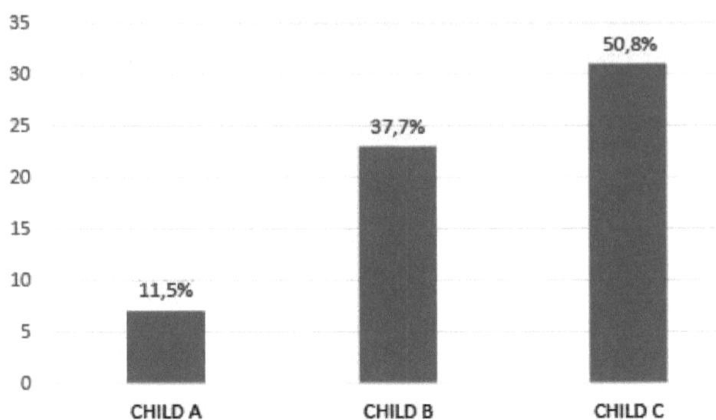

Figure 5: *Distribution of patients according to Child Pugh score*

1.3.3.2. MELD score

The median MELD score was14 [11-18]with extremes ranging from 6 to 39 (Figure 6).

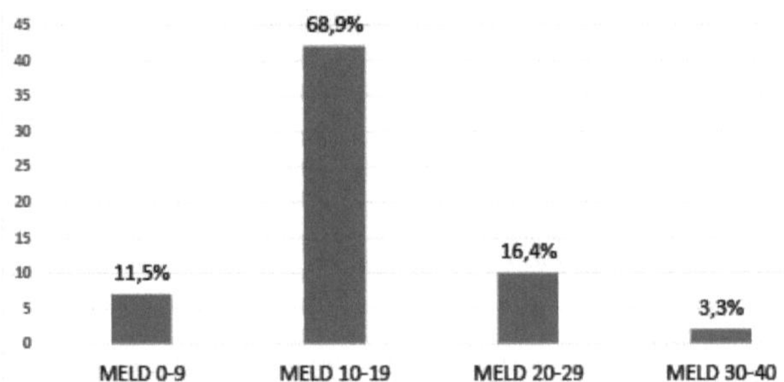

Figure 6. *Distribution according to MELD score*

It was greater than or equal to 15 in 28 patients (45.9%).

1.4. Characteristics of bacterial infections :

1.4.1. Site and type of infection :

The most frequent sites of bacterial infection diagnosed in our series were urinary, in 26 patients (42.6%), ascites fluid in 13 patients (21.3%) and bronchopulmonary in 8 patients (13.3%). UTI was associated with spontaneous ascites fluid infection in 1 patient (1.6%). Osteoarticular infection was observed in 3 patients (4.8%) (Table V).

Table V. *Different sites of infection*

Infection sites	Numbers (N=61)	Percentage (%)
IU	26	42,6
ILA	13	21,3
Bronchopulmonary infection	8	13,3

Infection of the ENT sphere	4	6,6
Erysipelas	4	6,6
Acute lithiasis angiocholitis	1	1,6
Complicated septic arthritis of the shoulder sepsis	1	16 1,6
Brucellosis spondylodiscitis	1	1,6
Lower genital infection	1	1,6
Pulmonary tuberculosis and osteoarticular	1 1	1 6 1,6
IU + ILA	1	1,6

Infection was community-acquired in 100% of patients (61

patients). There were no cases of healthcare-associated infection.

1.4.2. The germs involved :

Thirty-two germs were isolated from the various microbiological samples, representing 52.5% of bacterial infections. Only 30 antibiotic susceptibility tests (49.2% of cases) were performed.

The germ was identified in 66% of ECBU tests and 20% of PELA tests.

Brucella spondylodiscitis was ruled out on the basis of clinical and radiological data and positive Wright serology.

A positive *Mycobacterium tuberculosis* PCR on bronchial biopsies led to the diagnosis of pulmonary tuberculosis associated with Pott's disease.

Of the germs identified, 81.3% were BGN (26 patients), of which *Escherichia coli* (E. coli) was the predominant germ in 53.5% of cases.

PGCs were found in four patients (12.5%). (Table VI).

polymicrobial infections were observed in our series.

Table VI. *Incriminated germs according to the site of the bacterial infection.*

infection.

Location of documented infection	Germ involved	Number (%)
Urinary (N=20)	• *E. coli*	14 (43.9%)
	• *Klebsiella pneumoniae*	2 (6.5%) 1
	• *Pseudomonas aeruginosa*	(3.1%) 1
	• *Staphylococcus epidermis*	(3.1%) 1
	• *Enterobacter aerogenes*	(3.1%) 1
	• *Citrobacter koseri*	(3.1%)
Ascites (N=6)	• *E. coli*	1 (3,1%)

	• *Klebsiella pneumoniae* • *Staphylococcus aureus* • *Streptococcus pneumoniae* • *Salmonella enterica* • *Staphylococcus epidermis*	1 (3,1%) 1 (3,1%) 1 (3,1%) 1 (3,1%) 1 (3,1%)
Broncho-pulmonary (N=3)	• *Klebsiella pneumoniae* • Intracellular germs • *Mycobacterium* tuberculosis	1 (3,1%) 1 (3,1%) 1 (3,1%)
Osteoarticular (N=2)	• *Mycobacterium* tuberculosis • *Brucella*	1 (3,1%) 1 (3,1%)
Joint-onset septicaemia (N=1)	- *Staphylococcus aureus*	1 (3,1%)
IU+ILA (N=1)	- *E. coli*	1 (3,1%)

*The intracellular germ responsible for the bronchopneumonia could not be isolated from bacteriological samples, due to lack of resources, but was suspected on the basis of clinical and radiological evidence, or the lack of improvement with amoxicillin and clavulanic acid and improvement with macrolides.

**This is the same tuberculosis infection (pulmonary and spinal).

1.4.3. Sensitivity of isolated bacteria to antibiotics :

According to the results of the various antibiotic susceptibility tests, two of the germs incriminated (6.7%) were MRB bacteria. These were *Klebsiella pneumoniaeBLSEisolated* from the culture of an ECBU and methicillin-resistant *Staphylococcus aureus* (isolated from blood cultures). The other germs were sensitive to antibiotics (N=19, i.e. 63.3%). Sixteen were GNB (84.2%) and 3 were PGC (15.8%) (Figure 7).

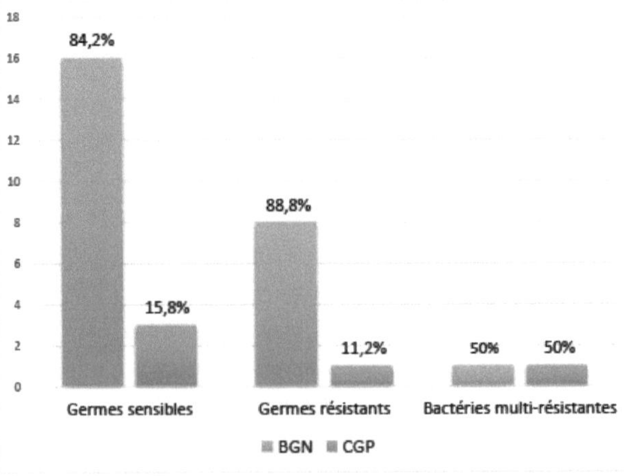

Figure 7. *The sensitivity of germs to antibiotics*

1.4.4. Characteristics the antibiotic therapy chosen :

Empirical 1st-line antibiotic therapy was administered to 57 patients (93%) as soon as the diagnosis was suspected and after the infectious disease investigation had been guided by clinical data.

In 11 cases (18%), this antibiotic therapy was modified after retrieving the antibiogram data.

Monotherapy was used in 88% of cases (n=54), dual therapy in 11% (n=6) and quadruple anti-tuberculosis therapy in only 1 patient.

The beta-lactam family was the most prescribed class (46 patients; 75%).

Among beta-lactam antibiotics, injectable C3G (Cefotaxime) was well ahead of other antibiotics (54%).

The median duration of antibiotic treatment was 10 days [5-12], with extremes ranging from 3 days to 15 months for pulmonary tuberculosis associated with Pott's disease.

1.5. qSOFA score on admission :

The qSOFA score was calculated retrospectively for all patients included in our study.

Forty-four percent of patients (n=27) had a score > 2, 93% of whom had a score equal to 2 and 7% of whom had a score equal to 3 (Figure 8).

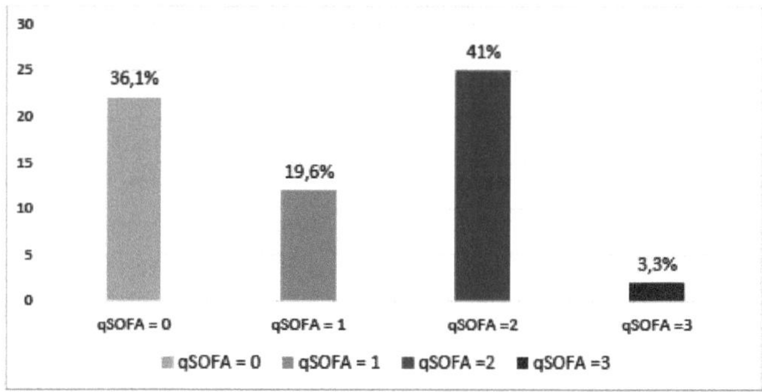

Figure 8. *Distribution of patients according to Qsofa score*

Among the parameters of the qSOFA score, aPAS<100mmHg was the most frequent, found in 25 patients (92.6%). Polypnoea was noted in 24 patients (88.9%).

Figure 9 shows the distribution of patients with a qSOFA score >2 according to the clinical parameters affected.

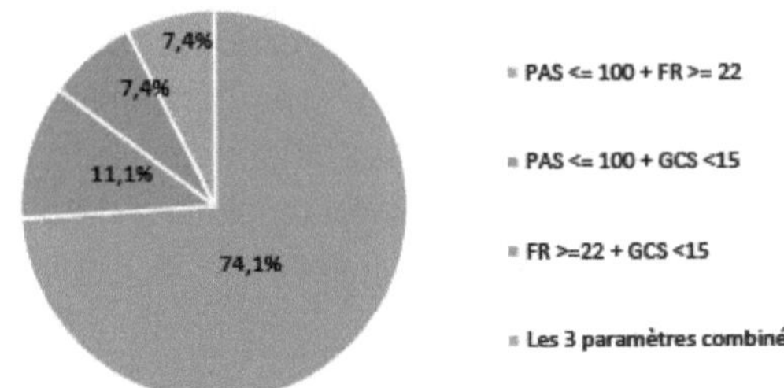

Figure 9. *Distribution of patients with a qSOFA score>2 according to clinical parameters*

9.6. Short-term trends :

9.6.1. In-hospital complications

Forty-six patients (75.4%) had a favourable outcome, judged by the disappearance of clinical symptoms in 45 patients (73.8%), resolution of SIB (n=45; 73.8%), culture negativation of a previously positive bacteriological examination (n=30; 49.2%) and radiological clearance (n=5; 8.2%), in the absence of complications, particularly haemodynamic and neurological, and in the absence of worsening of cirrhosis.

During hospitalisation, one or more complications occurred in 15 cirrhotics (25%) (table VII).

HE was the most frequent complication, occurring in 14 patients (23%), followed by the onset or worsening of IR (excluding hepato-renal syndrome (n=11; 18%).

Septic EDC was noted in 9 patients (14.8%), two of whom required transfer to a medical intensive care unit. Five patients had EDC with a urinary origin (*E. coli* (n=2), *Klebsiella pneumoniae* (n=1), unidentified germs (n=2) and 3 patients had EDC complicating an ALI (*Pneumococcus* (n=1) and unidentified germs (n=2). Another patient had CDE associated with a UTI associated with an ALI (*E. coli*).

ACLF was observed in 6 patients (9.8%).

Table VII. *In-hospital complications of bacterial infection*

Complication	Workforce	Percentage (%)
EH	14	23
Appearance or worsening an IR	11	18
EDC septic	9	14,8
Respiratory distress	7	11,5

***ACLF*6**	9,8

9.6.2. Complications and qSOFA score :

Of the 14 patients who developed a HAE complication after the infectious episode, 12 (85.7%) had a qSOFA >2.

Eight (88.9%) of the nine patients who developed septic DME had a qSOFA score >2.

The following table (Table VIII) shows the number of patients with a positive qSOFA according to the complications that occurred.

Table VIII. *In-hospital complications and qSOFA*

Complication	Number with qSOFA >2	Percentage (%)
EH	12	85,7
Onset or worsening of IR	9	81,8
EDC septic	8	88,9
Respiratory distress	6	85,7
ACLF	6	100

9.6.3. Length of hospital stay :

The median length of hospital stay was 18 days [10-25], with extremes ranging from 2 days to 52 days.

9.7. Mortality :

9.7.1. Overall mortality

Twenty-five deaths (41%) occurred during the study period. The median time to death was 30 days [0-315], with extremes ranging from 1 day, i.e. the same day as admission, to 1 year (Figure 10).

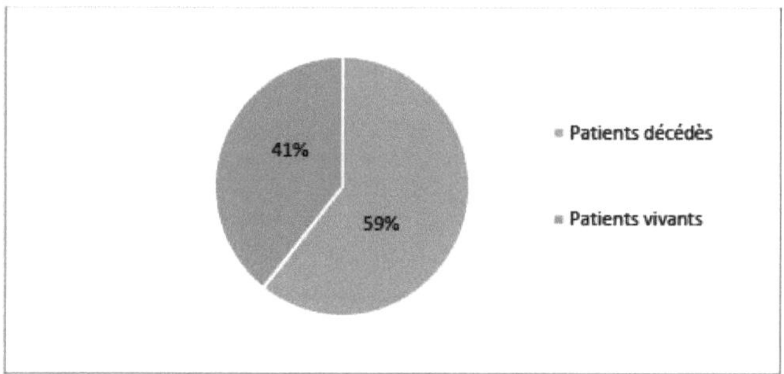

Figure 10. *Overall mortality*

The mean overall survival in our series was 161 months (95% CI between 112 months and 210 months) with a maximum survival of 336 months. The median survival was 108 months (Figure 11).

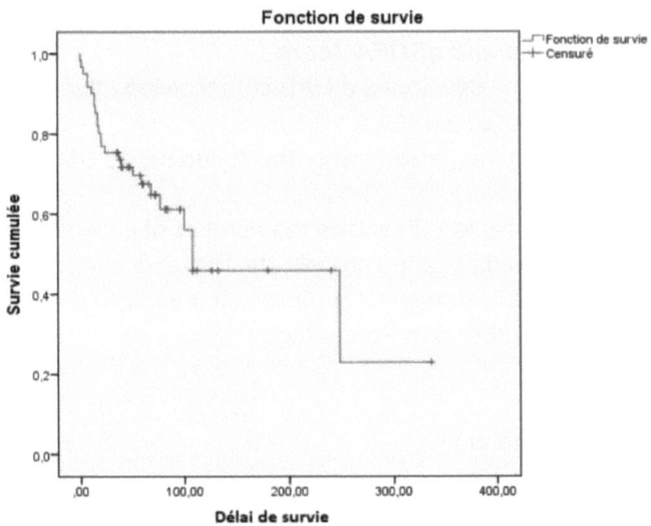

Figure 11. *Kaplan Meier survival curve for 61 patients*

1.7.2. In-hospital mortality

Ten patients (16%) died during their hospitalisation for bacterial infection. Death occurred, on average, after 10 days, with extremes ranging from 1 day to 25 days.

Of these patients who died in hospital, seven patients (70%) had an ALI (5 of whom were at the refractory ascites stage) and two patients (20%) had a UTI. (Figure 12).

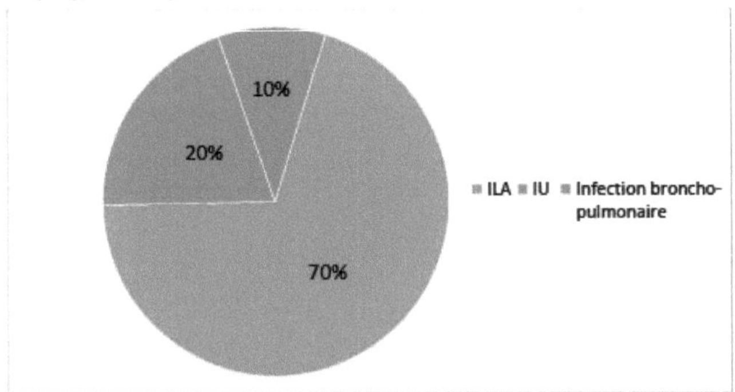

Figure 12. *In-hospital mortality by site of infection. infection.*

Seventy per cent of patients who died in hospital (n=7) CHILD C (figure 13).

Eight patients had a MELD >15 (80%). (Figure 14).

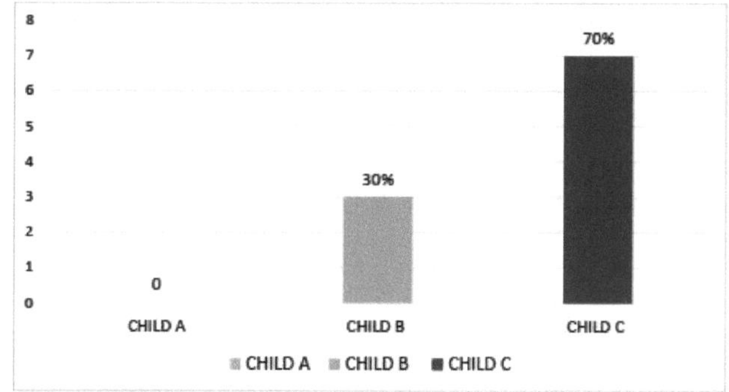

Figure 13. *In-hospital mortality as a function of CHILD*

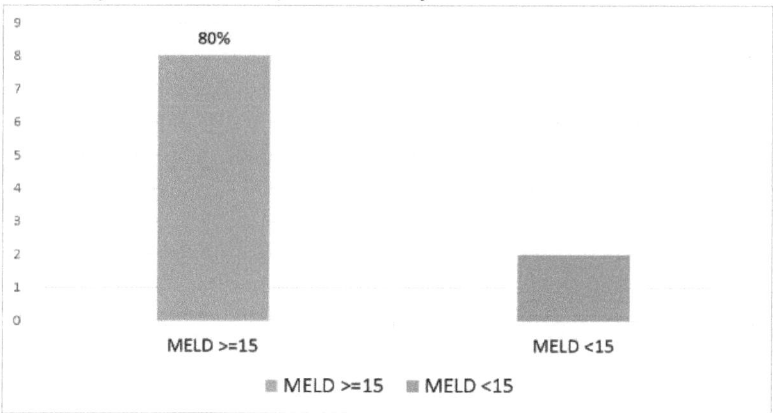

Figure 14. *In-hospital mortality as a function of MELD*

1.7.3. Mortality during follow-up

Fifteen patients (25%) died during the follow-up period, with an average delay of 224 days and extremes ranging from 14 days to 360 days. Eleven patients (18%) died within the first six months after hospitalisation, and four patients (6.6%) died between six and twelve months after hospital discharge. The most frequent infections in patients who died during follow-up were urinary (40%), bronchopulmonary (20%) and skin (20%) (Table IX).

Table IX. *Types of infection associated with mortality during follow-up*

Site of infection	Number of deaths	Percentage
IU	6	40%
Bronchopulmonary infection	3	20%

Erysipelas	3	20%
ILA	2	13%
IU+ ILA	1	7%

Of the patients who died after hospital discharge, 11 (79%) had a CHILD C score and 7 (46.7%) had a MELD > 15.

Of the patients who died within six months of hospital discharge, 9 (81.8%) CHILD C and 6 (54.5%) had MELD > 15 (Figures 15 and 16).

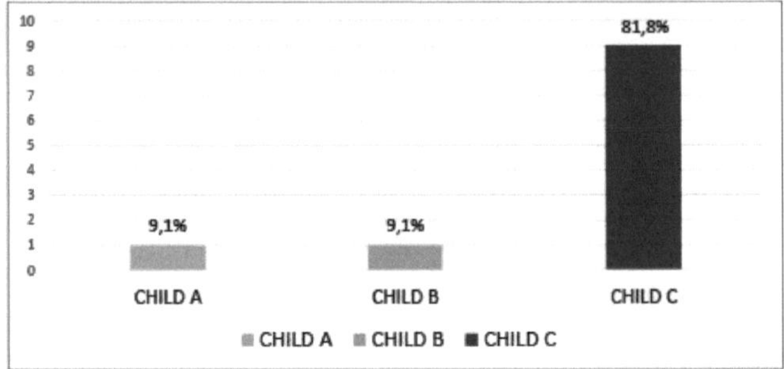

Figure 15. *Mortality at 6 months according to CHILD*

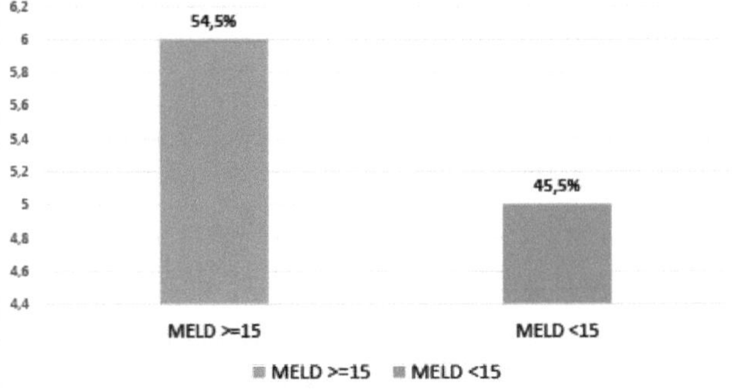

Figure 16. *Mortality at 6 months according to MELD*

Of the patients who died within 6-12 months of hospital discharge, 3 patients (75%) had a CHILD C score and 3 patients (75%) had a MELD < 15 (Figures 17 and 18).

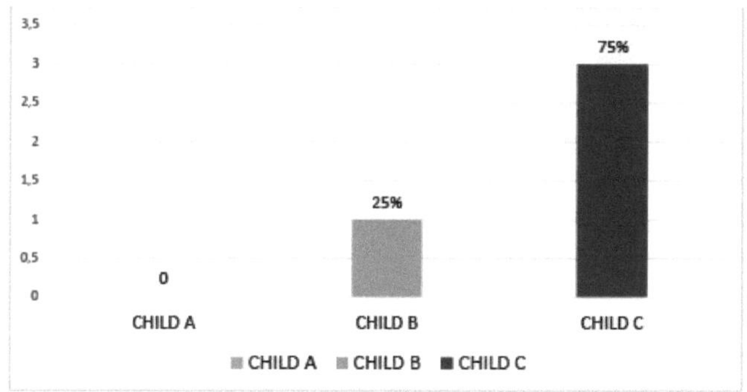

Figure 17. *Mortality at 12 months according to CHILD*

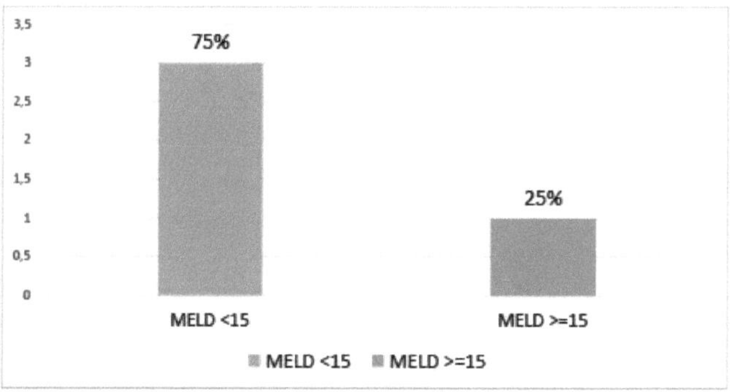

Figure 18. *Mortality at 12 months according to MELD*

1.7.4. Mortality according to qSOFA score :

Of the 25 patients who died, 24 (96%) had a qSOFA score > 2.

Within the hospital, nine (90%) of the ten cirrhotic patients who died had a score >2.

All patients who died during the follow-up period (n=15, 100%) had a score >2 (Figure 19).

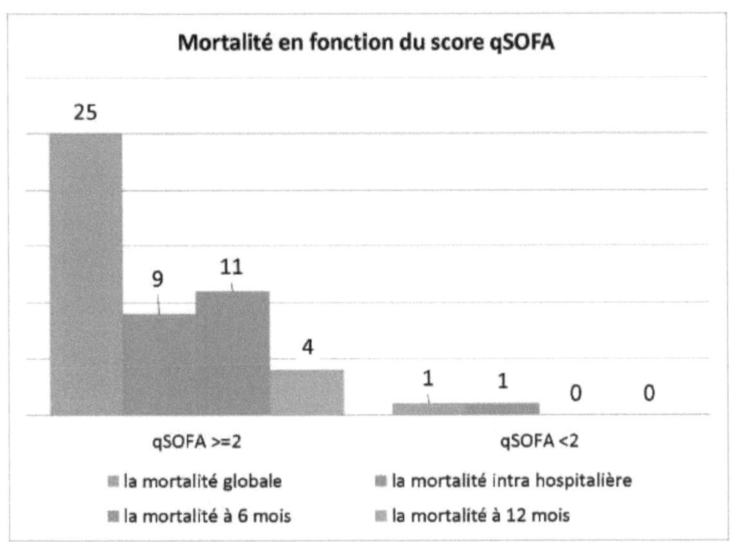

Figure 19. *Overall, in-hospital, 6-month and 12-month mortality by qSOFA score*

The mean survival in the group of patients with a qSOFA score <2 was 326 months (95% CI between 308 months and 344 months) and in the group with a score >2 was 60 months (95% CI between 31 months and 88 months) with a median of 24 months (Figure 20).

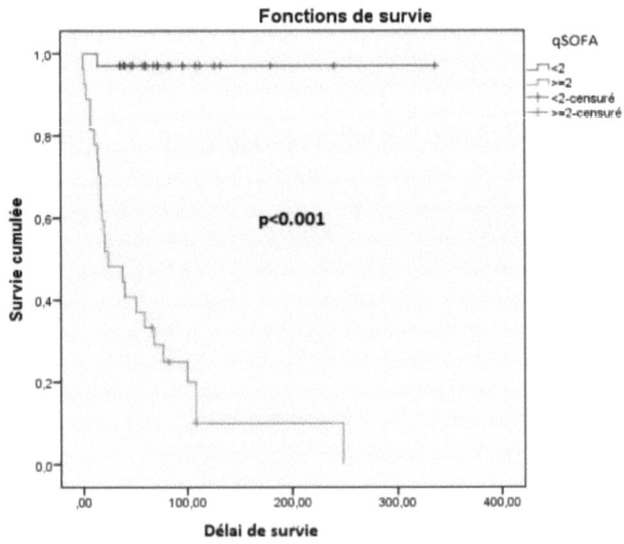

Figure 20: Kaplan Meier survival curve as a function of qSOFA score

The cumulative survival study showed a statistically significant difference between the two groups (**p<0.001**).

2. Analytical study :

2.1. Univariate analysis :

We carried out a univariate study of factors predictive of death in our population.

2.1.1. Factors associated with death other than the qSOFA score :

2.1.1.1. Analysis of patient characteristics and clinical data :

All parameters relating to the terrain and clinical examination data collected on admission were analysed. No parameters related to the terrain were associated with an increased risk of death.

Table X summarises the clinical examination data associated an increased risk of death

Table X. *Clinical parameters and mortality*

Parameter analysed	Workforce	Value of p
SAR<=100mm Hg	21	**<0.001**
Polypnoea	16	**0.032**
GCS <15	8	**0.004**
General state of health	16	**0.001**
DOA	24	**0.006**
EH	18	**<0.001**

2.1.2. Analysis of biological data :

All biological parameters relating to the infectious episode were analysed.

Hyperleukocytosis, elevated CRP and hyponatremia were associated with mortality with a **p=0.04**, **p=0.01** and **p=0.002**, respectively.

2.1.3. Bacterial infection :

The type of infection, the site and the germs involved were not associated with a high risk of mortality.

2.1.4. Analysis of cirrhosis characteristics :

CHILD-PUGH and MELD scores and the stage of refractory ascites were analysed.

The results are summarised in Table XI below:

Table XI. *CHILD and MELD scores and overall mortality*

Parameter	Workforce	Overall mortality
	CHILD	

CHILD A	1	0.127
CHILD B	5	**0.017**
CHILD C MELD score	19	**0.001**
MELD>15	15	0.06
MELD < 15	10	0.114
Refractory ascites stage	7	0.480

2.2. The qSOFA Score :

2.2.1. *Association of score with complications :*

The qSOFA score>2 was associated with an unfavourable outcome, according to the data from our study, with a significant risk **p=0.001**. Table XII below summarises the association of the score with the complications noted during the infectious episode:

Table XII. *qSOFA and complications*

Complication	Workforce	p
EH	12	0.844
Onset or worsening of IR	9	0.346
EDC septic	8	**0.035**
ACLF	6	**0.008**
Respiratory distress	6	0.064

A qSOFA score >2 was not associated with a longer hospital stay, according to our study (p=0.201).

2.2.2. *qSOFA and mortality :*

Of the 25 patients who died, 24 had a qSOFA score > 2, i.e. 96% of cases.

A score >2 was statistically significantly associated with overall mortality with a **p<0.001**.

Table XIII below shows the association between mortality and the qSOFA score

Table XIII. *qSOFA and mortality*

Mortality	Workforce	p
In-hospital	**9**	**0.078**
At 6 months	**11**	**0.366**
At 12 months	**4**	**0.656**

2.2.3. Analytical study: ROC curves for score performance :

2.2.3.1. qSOFA and overall mortality:

The AUROC for the qSOFA score was **0.953** (95% CI 0.899 - 1) (Figure).

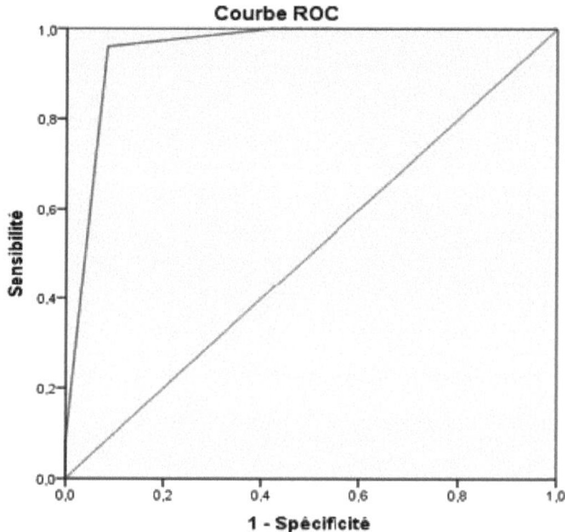

Figure 21: ROC curve of qSOFA score and overall mortality

2.2.3.2. qSOFA and in-hospital mortality at 6 and 12 months:

The AUROC for the qSOFA score was **0.550** (95% CI 0.300 - 0.800) for in-hospital mortality (Figure).

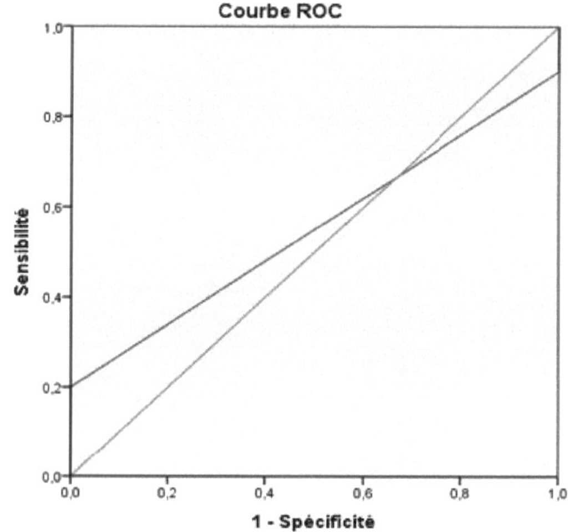

Figure 22: ROC curve of qSOFA score and in-hospital mortality

The AUROC for the qSOFA score was **0.524** (95% CI 0.237 - 0.810) for 6-month mortality.

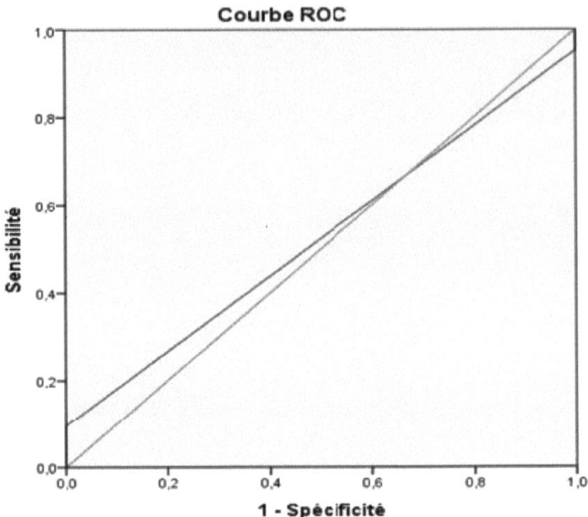

Figure 23: ROC curve of qSOFA score and 6-month mortality

The AUROC for the qSOFA score was **0.476** (95% CI 0.190 - 0.763) for mortality at 12 months (Figure).

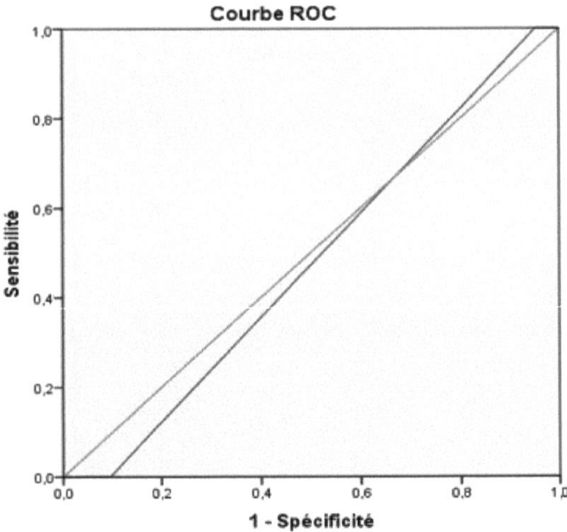

Figure 24: ROC curve of qSOFA score and mortality at 12 months

2.3. Multivariate analysis :

We carried out a multivariate study of factors predictive of death in our population.

The predictive factors for death that emerged in our study are summarised in the following table (Table XIV)

__Table XIV.__ Factors predictive of death

Predictive factor	Workforce	p
Development of an ACLF	6	<0.001
SGS < 15	8	<0.001
Development of an EDC	8	<0.001
General state of health admission	16	<0.001

4 DISCUSSION

We conducted a retrospective, descriptive study in the Gastroenterology-Hepatology B department at La Rabta to assess the qSOFA score in cirrhotic patients hospitalised for bacterial infection, the main cause of decompensation in cirrhosis.

To do this, we studied the epidemiological profile of bacterial infections in a Tunisian population of cirrhotic patients, calculated the qSOFA score retrospectively on admission and analysed the prognostic value of the score in this population in terms of complications and mortality over a 12-month period.

1. Main results :

During the study period, 61 eligible patients were hospitalised for bacterial infection complicating cirrhosis with a median duration progression of 24 months. Our population was predominantly female and the mean age at inclusion was 63 ±12 years. Smoking and alcohol consumption were noted in 26.2% and 3.3% of cirrhotic patients respectively. The main comorbidities were diabetes and hypertension, found in 20 (32.8%) and 16 (26.2%) patients respectively. Viral aetiology (HCV or HBV) was the predominant aetiology, observed in 63.9% of our patients. Infection was inaugural in 15% of cases. The main reason for consultation was AOD (78.8%), followed by abdominal pain (63.9%). Urinary signs were reported in 39.4% of cases. The average consultation time was 12 days. Physical examination revealed ascites and arterial hypotension in 86.9% and 55.7% of patients, respectively. Polypnoea and altered general condition were noted in 47.5% and 37.7% of cases, respectively. SIB was present in the majority of patients (80.3%) on laboratory tests. On admission, the majority of patients were classified as CHILD-PUGH C (50.8%) and 45.9% had a MELD score > 15. An infectious disease investigation was carried out in all patients. UTI (42.6%) and ALI (21.3%) were the most frequent. The infectious agent was identified in thirty-two patients (52.5%). BGN represented 81.3% of the germs isolated and *Escherichia coli* was the predominant infectious agent (53.1%). Empirical first-line antibiotic therapy was initiated in 93% of patients. It was mainly based on monotherapy (88%). Injectable C3Gs were the most commonly prescribed molecules (75%).

A positive qSOFA score (>2), calculated retrospectively, was present in 44% of patients. The median hospital stay was 18 days with a favourable outcome in 75.4% of cases. One or more complications were observed in 24.6% of patients. Hepatic encephalopathy was noted in 23% of infected cirrhotics, and progression to septic ED and ACLF was observed in 14.8% and 9.8% of patients, respectively. Forty-one per cent of cirrhotics died during the 12-month follow-up, with an in-hospital mortality rate of 16%. Twenty-four (96%) of the cirrhotic patients who died had a qSOFA score >2. In our study, a positive qSOFA score was significantly associated with the development of septic DCI and ACLF. Similarly, overall mortality was significantly higher in cirrhotic patients with a qSOFA score >2. Similarly, when analysing the ROC curves for qSOFA score and mortality, the area under the curve (AUROC) was 0.953, 0.550, 0.524 and 0.476 for overall, in-hospital, 6-month and 12-month mortality, respectively.

Prediction of mortality by univariate analysis revealed a significant association with the following clinical parameters: arterial hypotension, EH, altered general condition, GCS<15, polypnoea and DOA. Hyperleukocytosis, elevated CRP and hyponatremia were the biological factors significantly associated with death. In the multivariate analysis, only the development of ACLF, a GCS<15, the development of EDC and altered general condition were retained as independent factors predicting mortality.

2. The strengths and weaknesses of the study :

2.1. The strengths of our study :

The strengths of our study were :

-The management of bacterial infection followed the recommendations of the various learned societies, which reduced the risk bias during the statistical study.

-Our study is the first Tunisian study to focus exclusively on the prognostic value of the qSOFA score following an episode of bacterial infection in cirrhotic patients.

2.2. The weaknesses of our study :

However, our study has a number of limitations:

- The retrospective and monocentric nature of data collection
- The small number of patients studied reduces the statistical power of our results concerning factors predictive of death.
- The heterogeneity of the population studied in terms of the characteristics of cirrhosis.

3. Bacterial infections in cirrhotics :

3.1. Demographic characteristics

Our population consisted of 61 patients with an average age of 63±12 years. The group was predominantly female, with a sex ratio of 0.65. In

Tunisian studies of infections in cirrhotic patients[10,11] the mean age was 63 and 59 years respectively.
In other studies investigating the involvement of qSOFA in cirrhosis [1216], the population was predominantly male and the average age was also in the sixth decade.

3.2. Characteristics associated with cirrhosis

3.2.1. Etiologies of cirrhosis

Alcohol was the predominant aetiology [10,12,13,14] in the various series reported in the literature. Viral aetiology was present in only 5 to 20% of cases [10,12,13,14]. In our series, viral cirrhosis (C or B) was the most common. Alcohol was present in only 3.3% of cases. This finding may explained by the heterogeneous geographical distribution of cirrhosis aetiologies, which are dominated by alcoholic origin in Western countries [14,15].

3.2.2. Severity of cirrhosis :

In our study, Child-Pugh class C was predominant at the time of the infectious episode (51%). This is consistent with data in the literature[10-13,14]. The median MELD score in our series was 14 points. In a Swiss observational study by M. Müller et al [15] and the study by Kim et al [16] evaluating the qSOFA score in 186 and 1622 infected cirrhotics, respectively, the mean MELD was 15 points.

3.3. Characteristics of the infectious episode

3.3.1. Clinical features :

The predominant reason for consultation in our patients was abdominal distension associated with swelling of the lower limbs in relation to DOA (78.8%), followed by the appearance of abdominal pain (63.9%), asthenia (62.3%), fever (52.5%) and urinary signs (20%). The median consultation time was 8 days.
In the literature, the reasons for consultation and admission of infected cirrhotics varied from study to study. The most frequently reported clinical signs were oedemato-ascitic syndrome (34%), fever (21%) and HE (11%) [18]. Abdominal pain accounted for 49% of consultations in cases of ALI[19].
The diagnosis of bacterial infections in cirrhotic patients remains tricky because of the non-specificity and subtlety of the clinical signs[2]. This could explain the long delays in consultation observed in these patients.
In the literature, studies have focused mainly on ALI[20]. Signs of peritoneal irritation or systemic inflammation, such as fever, tachycardia and diarrhoea [19], generally dominate the clinical picture in patients

included in these studies.
In our series, the clinical examination revealed DOA in 78.8% of patients, fever in 36.1%, and an altered general condition in 37.7% of patients. The American study by Orman et al, which included 79092 cirrhotic patients and assessed their general condition, showed that 13% had an altered general condition. This group of patients had a significantly high overall mortality rate[21].

3.3.2. Biological characteristics :

Biological tests were performed on all our patients. The main abnormalities were anaemia (83.7%) and elevated CRP (80.3%). Hyperleukocytosis was noted in 24.6% of patients. Hyponatremia and IR were observed in 16.4% and 9.8% of cases, respectively.

In a meta-analysis [22], an elevated CRP (>29 mg/l) was found in 37.3% of patients. A wide variety of threshold values for CRP have been reported in the literature [23]. Authors tend to choose a higher threshold than is usual in the general population, given that CRP production by the liver is impaired in cirrhosis. In our study, we chose a threshold >10mg/l to define elevated CRP. This threshold was highly discriminatory in the study by Papp et al [24] (the AUROC of CRP was 0.93 with a sensitivity of 84% and a specificity of 91%).

Furthermore, according to our results, 83.7% of patients presented with anaemia. Anemia is observed in 75% of cirrhotics according to the literature [25] and is generally multifactorial (hypersplenism, haemorrhage, etc.).

This anaemia is all the more present and severe the more advanced the cirrhosis. Haemoglobin values are inversely proportional to the MELD score and are significantly lower in cirrhotics with a higher Child score[26].

In our series, the majority of infected cirrhotics were classified as Child C. The severity of liver disease could therefore explain the high prevalence of anaemia in the patients in our study.

Hyperleukocytosis, defined as a count > 10000 ele/mm3, was present in only 24.6% of our patients. This could be attributed to a "relative" rise in leukocyte count to normal values in these patients with leukopenia due to hypersplenism [27].

Furthermore, in cirrhotic patients, hyponatremia is significantly associated with a higher risk of mortality [9,25]. This biological parameter is widely sought in prognostic studies of cirrhotic patients, particularly infected cirrhotics [8,28]. We diagnosed hyponatremia in 16.4% of our patients. In the Tunisian studies cited above, hyponatremia was noted in almost half of infected cirrhotics, i.e. in 48% of patients [10], and in approximately one-third of patients (29.9%) in the study by Houissa et al[9]. In the latter study, hyponatremia was significantly correlated with death (p=0.049).

IR was noted in only 10% of our patients. In a prospective Italian study evaluating IR in infected cirrhotic patients, it was 23% in patients without ascites versus 59% in patients with ascites[29]. The low prevalence of IR in our series could be explained by the non-inclusion of patients with SHR and the exclusion of those who developed this complication during follow-up.

3.3.3. Microbiological characteristics

In our series, the germ responsible for the infection was isolated in 52.5% of cases. In the literature[8,30], a germ was isolated in almost two-thirds of infections. BGN were the germs most frequently incriminated in the patients in our study, with *Escherichia coli* the most frequently identified infectious agent, in 53.5% of patients.

PGCs were found in 12.5% of cases. These data are consistent with the literature. BGN remain the predominant germs, causing more than half of all infections (53%). *Escherichia* coli was present in 2/3 of infections according to various studies [14,27,29]. CGPs were implicated in 39% of cases [30]. In our study, BMR were found in only 2 patients (7%). These were an ESBL-secreting *Klebsiella pneumoniae* and a methicillin-resistant *Staphylococcus aureus*. In the literature, the overall prevalence of BMR in cirrhotic infections is 34%[13,31], a figure much higher than ours. This could be explained by the small number of our patients, the bacteriological profile of germs depending on the site of infection [32,33] and the bacterial ecosystem, which is specific to each hospital department [34].

3.3.4. Seat of infection :

Based on the results of our study, urinary tract infections accounted for 42.6% of all bacterial infections, followed by ALI and bronchopulmonary infections, which were found in 21.3% and 13.3% of our patients, respectively. These values are consistent with a Tunisian retrospective study [11] evaluating the factors predictive of mortality in 97 infected cirrhotics. The infections identified were, in order of frequency, urinary (38%), ascitic (30%), bronchopulmonary, cutaneous and gynaecological.

In the literature, and particularly in a multicentre French study [30] that included 1093 cirrhotic patients, ALI was the most common infection

(29%), followed by urinary tract infection (20%) and bronchopulmonary infection (17%). These results concur with those of a prospective, multicentre study by Piano S et al [13].

3.4. Antibiotic therapy

Probabilistic intravenous antibiotic therapy was prescribed immediately after appropriate microbiological samples were taken from all our patients. This prescription was subsequently adapted to the results of the samples. Our therapeutic management was fully in line with the recommendations of learned societies [8].

Indeed, any delay in initiating antibiotic treatment is associated with a higher mortality rate [35]. The choice of probabilistic antibiotic therapy should therefore depend on the site and severity of the infection, and on the microbiological profile of hospital and community-acquired germs [8,35]. In our study, the beta-lactam family was the most commonly used class (75%). Injectable C3Gs (cefotaxime) were well ahead of other antibiotics, prescribed as mono- or dual therapy in 54% of cases. The duration of treatment depended on the nature of the infection and subsequent course. The median duration in our series was 10 days.

For many years, injectable C3Gs were considered the gold standard in the treatment of infections in cirrhotic patients. This is because C3Gs are active against enterobacteriaceae and non-enterococcal streptococci, the germs most often implicated in urinary tract infections and LAI in cirrhotic patients [36]. Furthermore, this class is generally well tolerated [37].

4. Complications and evolution

4.1. Length of hospital stay

The average length of hospitalisation was 19 days. These results are in line with a retrospective Tunisian study of infected cirrhotics, where the average length of hospitalisation was also 19 days [11].

In the literature, the average length of hospitalisation during an infectious episode in cirrhotic patients varies. It is estimated at 15 days in a Portuguese study [38] and 4 days in an American study [3]. In the Swiss study by M. Müller et al [15] and the study by Kim et al [16], the average length of hospitalisation was 8 days.

4.2. Short-term evolution and in-hospital complications

In our series, HE was the most frequent complication, occurring in 14 patients (23% of cases). In an Italian study, this complication was observed in 79% of cases[13]. IR was observed in 18% of our patients. In the literature, one third of infected cirrhotic patients develop functional

IR[39], which is of prerenal origin and due to a decrease in renal blood flow following arterial vasodilatation of the splanchnic and systemic territories. It remains the most common cause, and renal function is often improved by simple vascular filling [40]. Nine patients in our series (14.8%) had developed septic DCI, 2 of whom required transfer to a medical intensive care unit. This figure is consistent with the international multicentre study by Piano S et al. In this series, thirteen per cent of bacterial infections were complicated by septic EDC[13]. In cirrhotic patients, the average incidence of severe sepsis is estimated at 4.5% per year. This incidence is five times higher than in the general population and is essentially associated with the severity of cirrhosis [41]. ACLF was observed in 9.8% of our patients. This complication was noted in 37% of patients in the European multicentre study by Moreau et al[42], involving 1343 cirrhotics. According to the literature, bacterial infections are associated with an increased risk of progression to ACLF and multi-organ failure[42,43].

4.3. Mortality :

In our series, mortality concerned 41% of patients, 40% of whom died in hospital and 60% during the 12-month follow-up after the infectious episode. Based on data from other studies

Tunisian[11], the intra-hospital mortality rate was 30.9%, twice that observed in our study. Septic shock (56.7%) and multi-visceral failure were the direct causes of death.

In a large review of the literature by Arvaniti et al [44] including 178 studies published between 1978 and 2009 and involving 11,987 cirrhotic patients, the authors found that the occurrence of an infection in these patients quadrupled the mortality rate, with rates of around 31.5% and 66.2% at one month and 12 months, respectively. This study highlighted the alarming fact that almost half of cirrhotic patients who survive sepsis will die within a year. Consequently, effective, rapid and early management is a real survival issue for infected cirrhotic patients.

The table below summarises the data in the literature concerning the in-hospital mortality rate and one-month follow-up in cirrhotic patients following an infection.

Table XV. *Intra-hospital mortality rate in infected cirrhotics infected cirrhotics in the various studies using the qSOFA score*

Study	Total population (n)	Number of patients who died	Mortality (%)

Our study	61	10	16,4
M. Müller et al **[15]**	186	29	15,6
Augustinho and al.**[14]**	382	45	27
Piano S et al **[12]**	259	45	17
Piano S et al. **[13]**	1302	293	23
Kim et al. **[16]**	1622	244	15

5. Prognosis score qSOFA

5.1. Interest of the qSOFA score in infected cirrhotics

It is well recognised that the SRIS criteria (Appendix 5) for the diagnosis of sepsis are imprecise in patients with cirrhosis and bacterial infections [12]. Indeed, cirrhotic patients may present with leukopenia due to hypersplenism, tachypnoea due to hepatic encephalopathy or the presence of ascites, and bradycardia due to the increasingly widespread prescription of beta-blockers to prevent digestive haemorrhage.

In 2016, a group of experts introduced new diagnostic criteria for the definition of sepsis in the general population. Sepsis is now defined as the combination of infection, host response and organ dysfunction [9]. The qSOFA score was developed in the context of this consensus. It is the most recent score recommended for the management of infected patients. One point is awarded each time the SCG is less than or equal to 15, the PAS is less than or equal to 100 mmHg and the RF is greater than or equal to 22. The sum of the points determines the qSOFA score. This new score, which does not take biological data into account in its calculation, appears to be a simple and rapid way of identifying patients at risk of developing sepsis. Nevertheless, the use of this score to assess prognosis in patients with cirrhosis and bacterial infection remains low[10,12,14].

5.2. qSOFA score on admission :

In our study, 44% of our patients (n=27) had a score greater than or equal to 2, i.e. a positive score. The table below compares the results of our study with those of studies conducted on infected cirrhotic patients with a positive qSOFA score on admission.

Table XVI. *Patients with a positive qSOFA on admission in the different series*

Study	Number of employees (n)	qSOFA >2 n (%)
Our study	61	25 (44%)
M. Müller et al[15].	186	22 (12%)
F.de Augustinho e al. [14]	164	33 (20%)
Piano S et al. [12]	259	60 (23%)
Piano S et al. [13]	1302	255 (23%)
Kim et al. [16]	1622	231 (14,2%)

We note that the percentage of patients with a positive score on admission in our series is almost double that observed in the literature. Despite the similarities between our population and those of these recent studies in terms of patient demographics (age, comorbidities) and severity of liver disease (CHILD and MELD scores), no explanation can be given. One possible reason could be a longer delay in consultation for our patients (a median delay of 8 days). Although the consultation time was not specified in these series.

5.3. Performance of the qSOFA score in infected cirrhotics The qSOFA score > was associated with an unfavourable outcome, according to the data from our study, with a significant risk **(p=0.001).** Indeed, the development of ACLF or septic EDC in patients with a positive score is increased with a p-value equal to **0.008** and **0.035**, respectively. This result is in line with that of the Italian multicentre series by Piano S et al[12,13]. These two prospective studies highlighted the proven role of this clinical score in identifying infected cirrhotic patients at risk of complications. Management in an appropriate intensive care setting is therefore necessary.

In our series, of the 25 patients who died, 24 had a qSOFA score > 2, i.e. 96% of cases. Statistical analysis showed that a positive score was significantly correlated with high overall mortality (**p < 0.001**) with an area under the ROC curve of **0.953**, demonstrating good sensitivity, without being a predictive factor of in-hospital mortality (**p=0.078**) or having a good performance as demonstrated by the AUROC of the score at **0.550** (95% CI 0.300 - 0.800). Similarly, this score was not correlated with medium- and long-term mortality (**p=0.366** and **p=0.656**, respectively).

In the study by Augustinho et al [14], the AUROC of the qSOFA score for overall mortality was 0.820 (95% CI 0.717 - 0.923). In the study by Kim et al [16], the AUROC of the qSOFA score was 0.67 (0.64-0.70) for in-hospital mortality, with a sensitivity of 39.6% and a specificity of 86.7%. For mortality at 1 month and 3 months it was 0.63 (0.61-0.66) and 0.60 (0.57-0.63), respectively.

No study in the literature has examined the long-term value of this score in infected cirrhotic patients. In-hospital mortality and one-month follow-up have been assessed [10-13,14]. Of the patients who died in our series, only one died at one month's follow-up, after discharge from hospital.

In the series by Kim et al [16], mortality was assessed over a 3-month follow-up. The results of this study showed that the qSOFA score not only had a predictive value for in-hospital mortality ($p<0.001$) and 1-month mortality ($p<0.001$), but also for 3-month follow-up ($p<0.001$).

According to the same study, the qSOFA score had a specificity of 86.7% in predicting in-hospital mortality, surpassing that of CLIF-SOFA (78.7%) and Sepsis-3 (74.8%). However, this score had the lowest sensitivity (36.6%) compared with the other scores.

In the same Tunisian series reported previously [11], the qSOFA score on admission was calculated. This score was significantly higher in patients who died than in those who survived. In the literature, and as already mentioned, re-evaluation of this score in cirrhotic patients following infection has been the subject of very few studies [12,14].

In the literature [10-12,14], this score was significantly associated with in-hospital mortality and short-term mortality, defined as mortality within 30 days of admission. These studies demonstrated the superiority of this score compared with the SRIS, which is widely used to predict mortality in infected cirrhotic patients. According to the authors of these studies, the SRIS no longer constitutes a prognostic score for evaluating infected cirrhotic patients. In fact, this score reflects an appropriate response to infection and no longer meets the new definition of sepsis[9]. Sepsis now represents a deregulated response by the body and could lead to organ dysfunction, a direct cause death following infection.

Furthermore, in the Brazilian study by Augustinho et al[14], when the qSOFA score was negative (< 2) on admission, the prognosis of patients was strongly linked to the occurrence of organ dysfunction complicating the infectious episode. Patients should therefore be carefully assessed within the first 48 hours (H48) of admission. If the qSOFA becomes greater than or equal to 2, at H48, and/or if the patient develops ACLF, hospitalisation in intensive care is recommended. The survival rate for patients transferred to the intensive care unit was 48% compared with 24% for non-transferred patients with a positive score and/or ACLF at H48 on admission. The same study proposed an algorithm for estimating the severity of infection in decompensated cirrhotic patients hospitalised for bacterial infection, based on the qSOFA score. This algorithm is shown in the figure below.

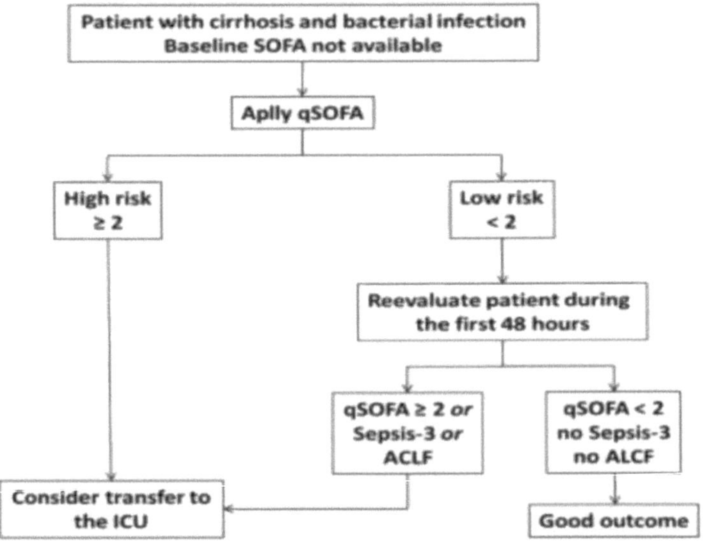

Figure 25. *Suggested algorithm for assessing the severity of infection in cirrhotic patients with a negative qSOFA on admission [14].*

In the Swiss study by M. Müller et al[15], qSOFA was not correlated with mortality (p=0.755), admissions to intensive care (p=0.152) or length of hospitalisation (p=0.489) in decompensated cirrhotic patients. The authors of this study evaluated this score in decompensated cirrhotic patients with and without infection. The authors believe that decompensated cirrhotic patients may share a certain pathophysiological similarity with infected non-cirrhotic patients with sepsis. The qSOFA could therefore, by analogy, be of prognostic interest in decompensated patients. However, the above-mentioned results did not support this hypothesis. The predictive performance proven for the general population [7] cannot be applied to a specific subgroup of patients, in this case decompensated cirrhotic patients. The qSOFA seems to be a less effective prognostic score in terms of cirrhosis decompensation. It would be more appropriate and relevant in the case infection.

We also note that in our series, the qSOFA score appears to be associated with short-term mortality. In the analytical study, the longer the follow-up time, the higher the "p" value and therefore the lower its statistical value (p=0.078 in the in-hospital setting, p=0.366 at 6 months and p=0.656 at 12 months).

In the light of all the above, the qSOFA score, which is a purely clinical score, has its place in the emergency department by enabling early detection of patients at high risk of mortality and complications. This could reduce the time taken to prescribe antibiotic therapy for these patients.

In 2018, at a meeting of European experts [8], a new algorithm was validated concerning the value of the qSOFA score and Sepsis- 3 (Appendix 6) in the management of infected cirrhotic patients. This algorithm, shown in Figure 22, was proposed by Piano S et al in the study described previously [12].

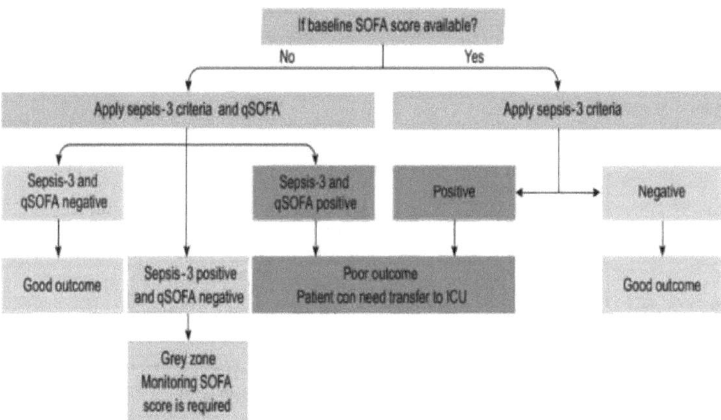

Figure 26. *Algorithm for application of qSOFA and Sepsis-3 scores in infected cirrhotics*

6. Factors associated with death other than the qSOFA score :

Apart from qSOFA, several factors associated with death have been reported in the literature.

Various series[12-15], like our own, have shown that DOA and EH are the two factors consistently associated with death.

Infection is a determining factor in the evolution of cirrhosis, either by causing decompensation of the disease or by grafting onto an already decompensated and advanced cirrhosis[43]. This could explain the latter finding.

The various clinico-biological factors predictive of mortality found in our series and in the literature are summarised in the following tables.

Table XVII. *Clinical parameters associated with death*

Study	Clinical parameters	p
	PAS<=100mm Hg	**<0.001**
	Polypnoea	**0.032**
Our study	GCS <15	**0.004**
	General state of health	**0.001**
	DOA	**0.006**
	EH	**<0.001**
Augustinho et al.	DOA	**<0.001**
[14]	EH	**0.003**
	DOA	0.159
	EH	**0.002**
Piano S et al *[12]*	Polypnoea	**0.001**
	Arterial hypotension	0.363
	DOA	**<0.001**
	EH Polypnoea	**<0.001**
Piano S et al *[13]*		**<0.001**
	Arterial hypotension	**<0.001**
M. Müller et al.	DOA Ictere EH	0.371
[15]		0.657
		0.294
Kim et al *[16]*	DOA	**0.02**
	EH	**<0.001**

Table XVIII. *Biological parameters associated with death*

Study	Biological parameters	P
	CRP	**0.01**
Our study	Hyponatremia	**0.002**
	Hyperleukocytosis	**0.04**
	CRP	**<0.001**
	Hyperleukocytosis Elevated	**0.027**
F.de Augustinho	creatinine	**<0.001**

***et al** [14]*	INR	**<0.001**
	Hyponatremia	**0.025**
	CRP	**0.019**
	Hypoalbuminemia	**0.012**
***Piano S et al** [12]*	High creatinine	**0.021**
	INR	**<0.001**
	Hyponatremia	**0.002**
	CRP	0 051
***Piano S et al** [13]*	Hyperleukocytosis	**<0.001**
	High creatinine	**0.001**
	INR	**<0.001**
	Hyponatremia	**<0.001**
	CRP	**<0.001**
	Hyperleukocytosis	**<0.001**
***Kim et al**[16]*	Hyponatremia	**<0.001**
	INR	**<0.001**

We note that the biological parameters most implicated in the mortality of infected cirrhotics, found in the various studies in the literature, are consistent with our results. An interesting point to note is that in the Swiss series from the University Centre of Bern by M. Müller et al [15], the authors adopted the qSOFA-Na+ score. In this study, qSOFA was increased by one point for admission serum sodium <130mmol/l. This biological parameter increased the predictive performance of qSOFA with regard to admission to intensive care (**p=0.001**) and in-hospital mortality (**p=0.038**).

With regard to cirrhosis severity scores, according to the studies, a high Child Pugh C and/or MELD score was associated with a high risk of mortality in infected cirrhotics. In series published in the literature [13,14], the authors chose a threshold >15 to define an advanced MELD score. This threshold was >21 points in the multicentre study by Piano et al [11].

In our study, we adopted a threshold > 15 to define advanced MELD. This threshold corresponds to the determining value in cirrhotic patients who are candidates for liver transplantation [45].

Comparing these scores with qSOFA, their prognostic value in terms of short-term mortality, according to the literature [4,5] and the results of our study, remains superior to qSOFA. Nevertheless, a meta-analysis would be necessary to reinforce this hypothesis. The table below summarises the results of these studies.

Table XIX. *Association of cirrhosis severity scores with mortality*

Study	**Severity score**	**P**
	CHILD C	**0.001**
Our study	MELD > 15	0.06
Augustinho et al.	CHILD C	**<0.001**
	*[14]*Advanced MELD	**<0.001**
Piano S et al *[12]*	CHILD C	**<0.001**
	Advanced MELD	**<0.001**
	CHILD C	**<0.001**
Piano S et al *[13]*	MELD> 21	**<0.001**
	CHILD C	0 880
M. Müller et al *[15]*	MELD> 15	**0.003**
	CHILD C MELD >15	**<0.001**
Kim et al *[16]*		**<0.001**

7. Tunisian theses on the subject :

When we searched the libraries of Tunisian medical faculties, we found no theses on the subject.

The only thesis to look at prognostic scores in cirrhosis concerned cirrhosis complicated HDH. In this work, the authors used the SOFA rather than the qSOFA.

In fact, the SOFA score and its simplified version qSOFA would be better assessed in infected cirrhotics admitted to liver intensive care units. The lack of such intensive care facilities in our country precludes such studies.

8. Proposed algorithm for the management of bacterial infection in cirrhotic patients based on the qSOFA score:

At the end of this work, we will be able to propose the following algorithm for the management of bacterial infection in cirrhotic patients, based on the qSOFA score and the severity of cirrhosis.

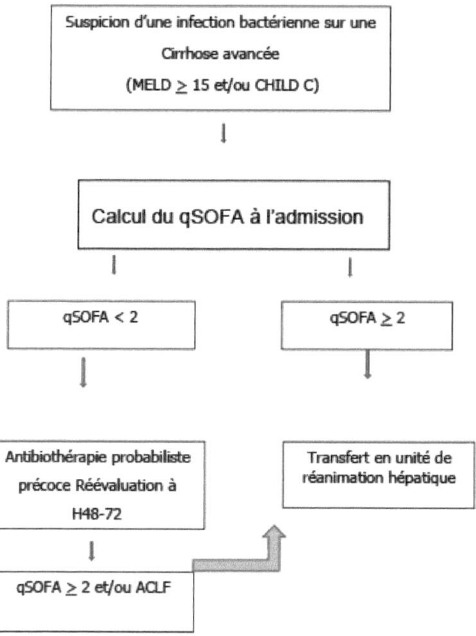

Figure 27. *Proposed algorithm for the management of cirrhotic patients with infected patients*

5 CONCLUSIONS

Bacterial infections are a late complication of cirrhosis, occurring in patients with advanced and usually decompensated liver disease.

A marker of severity, they also contribute to the deterioration of already impaired liver function, and the risk death from sepsis is particularly high.

Consequently, early identification and prompt management of cirrhotic patients with bacterial infection is vital.

The qSOFA score, established in 2016, has shown good diagnostic performance, can be used in emergency departments during the management of sepsis and does not differ significantly from other more complex scores. In fact, this score is proving useful for screening for organ failure in patients with suspected infection. It comprises 3 easily measurable clinical variables (PAS <100, FR >22, GCS<15). A positive score (>2) is predictive of sepsis mortality in the general population.

However, this purely clinical score has not been sufficiently evaluated in infected cirrhotic patients and the results are heterogeneous between series, hence the aim of our study to evaluate the relevance of this score, established on admission, in predicting mortality in cirrhotic patients with bacterial infection.

We conducted a descriptive, retrospective study in the Gastroenterology-Hepatology B Department of the Rabta Hospital over a five-year period, from January 2016 to December 2020, including 61 cirrhotic patients admitted for bacterial infection.

Cirrhotic patients with a history of progressive neoplastic pathology other than HCC and/or who had, at inclusion, an episode of HDH, SHR and/or HCC were not included in the study. Patients who were lost to follow-up and whose records could not be retrieved were excluded. Similarly, cirrhotic patients who presented a second episode of bacterial infection or a complication such as HDH and/or SHR and/or HCC during the study period were excluded.

Data were collected from medical records. For each patient included, we calculated the qSOFA score on admission and assessed the performance of this score in terms of mortality and complications.

Mortality was assessed using survival curves based on the Kaplan Meier model, and sensitivity and specificity were studied using ROC curves and areas under the ROC curve (AUROC). As for complications, we carried out a univariate and multivariate study a logistic regression model.

For all statistical tests, a p-value is significant if less than 0.05.

During the study period, we enrolled 61 patients with a mean age of 63±12 years and a gender ratio of 0.65 men to women.

Diabetes and hypertension, found respectively in 20 (32.8%) and 16 (26.2%) patients, were the most frequent comorbidities.

Viral aetiology of cirrhosis (HCV or HBV) was predominant aetiology in 63.9% of our patients, with a median duration of disease progression of 24 months.

Infection was inaugural in 15% of cases.

DOA was the main reason for consultation (78.8%).

majority of patients were classified as CHILD-PUGH C (50.8%) and 45.9% had a MELD score > 15.

Urinary tract infection and spontaneous ascites infection were the predominant infections (42.6% and 21.3% respectively).

Thirty-two germs were isolated, with BGN accounting for 81.3% and *Escherichia coli* being

the predominant germ in 53.5% of cases.
Injectable C3Gs were most commonly used antibiotic therapy molecules (54%).
A positive qSOFA score (>2) was present in 44% of patients.
The median hospital stay was 19 days, with a favourable outcome in 75% of cases.
Forty-one per cent of infected cirrhotics died after the infectious episode and during the 12-month follow-up.
Of the 25 patients who died, 24 (96%) had a qSOFA score >2.
The analytical study showed several factors predictive of death apart from qSOFA; the clinical parameters included arterial hypotension, EH, impaired general condition, GCS <15, polypnoea and DOA. Hyperleukocytosis, elevated CRP and hyponatremia were the biological factors significantly associated with death.
In our study, the qSOFA score was predictive of the occurrence of complications, and therefore of an unfavourable outcome (p=0.001) such as the development of septic DCI and ACLF, with p values of 0.035 and 0.008, respectively, and of overall mortality (p<0.001). For in-hospital mortality, the p-value was close to the significance level (**p=0.078**). This was in contrast to medium- and long-term mortality, for which the p-values were equal to 0.366 and 0.656, respectively.
Mean survival in cirrhotic patients with a qSOFA score <2 was significantly higher than in patients with a positive score >2 (326 versus 60 months).
The cumulative survival study showed a statistically significant difference between the two groups (**p<0.001**).
The ROC curves for the qSOFA score and mortality showed areas under the curve of 0.953, 0.550, 0.464 and 0.476 for overall, intra-hospital, 6-month and 12-month mortality, respectively. Consequently, the specificity and sensitivity of the qSOFA score for predicting mortality was higher in terms of overall mortality over a 12-month follow-up.
In view of our results, the qSOFA score has an important prognostic value in predicting the occurrence of intra-hospital complications and overall mortality over a 12-month follow-up.
This prognostic value seems to be less and less important in terms of mortality occurring at a distance from the infectious episode, i.e. in the medium and long term.
The main limitations of our study are the retrospective, monocentric nature and the small number of patients in our series, which reduced the statistical power of the study.
Given the simplicity of its calculation, it would be judicious to consider qSOFA in the early management of infected cirrhotics, from the time of admission.
Prospective studies on a larger scale would be interesting to confirm these results.
In Tunisia, we have a terrible shortage of liver resuscitation services, and setting up these intensive care facilities could improve the survival of infected cirrhotics.

6 BIBLIOGRAPHY

[1] Fernández J, Navasa M, Gómez J, Colmenero J, Vila J, Arroyo V, et al. Bacterial infections in cirrhosis: Epidemiological changes with invasive procedures and norfloxacin prophylaxis: Bacterial Infections in Cirrhosis: Epidemiological Changes With Invasive Procedures and Norfloxacin Prophylaxis. Hepatology 2002;35:140-8. https://doi.Org/10.1053/jhep.2002.30082.

[2] Deutsch M, Manolakopoulos S, Andreadis I, Giannaris M, Kontos G, Kranidioti H, et al. Bacterial infections in patients with liver cirrhosis: clinical characteristics and the role of C-reactive protein. Ann Gastroenterol 2018;31:77-83. https://doi.org/10.20524/aog.2017.0207.

[3] Desai AP, Mohan P, Nokes B, Sheth D, Knapp S, Boustani M, et al. Increasing Economic Burden in Hospitalized Patients With Cirrhosis: Analysis of a National Database. Clin Transl Gastroenterol 2019;10:e00062. https://doi.org/10.14309/ctg.0000000000000062.

[4] Coxeter-Smith C, Al-Adhami A, Alrubaiy L. The Usefulness of Mayo End-stage Liver Disease (MELD) and MELD-Sodium (MELD-Na) Scores for Predicting Mortality in Cirrhotic Patients With Spontaneous Bacterial Peritonitis. Cureus 2023. https://doi.org/10.7759/cureus.38343.

[5] Peng Y, Qi X, Guo X. Child-Pugh Versus MELD Score for the Assessment of Prognosis in Liver Cirrhosis: A Systematic Review and Meta-Analysis of Observational Studies. Medicine 2016;95:e2877. https://doi.org/10.1097/MD.0000000000002877.

[6] Rashed E, Soldera J. CLIF-SOFA and CLIF-C scores for the prognostication of acute-on-chronic liver failure and acute decompensation of cirrhosis: A systematic review. World J Hepatol 2022;14:2025-43. https://doi.org/10.4254/wjh.v14.i12.2025.

[7] Singer AJ, Ng J, Thode HC, Spiegel R, Weingart S. Quick SOFA Scores Predict Mortality in Adult Emergency Department Patients With and Without Suspected Infection. Ann Emerg Med 2017;69:475-9. https://doi.org/10.1016/j.annemergmed.2016.10.007.

[8] European Association for the Study of the Liver. Electronic address: easloffice@easloffice.euEuropean Association for the Study of the Liver. EASL Clinical Practice Guidelines for the management of patients with decompensated cirrhosis. J Hepatol 2018;69:406-60. https://doi.org/10.1016/jJhep.2018.03.024.

[9] Singer M, Deutschman CS, Seymour CW, Shankar-Hari M, Annane D, Bauer M, et al. The Third International Consensus Definitions for Sepsis and Septic Shock (Sepsis-3). JAMA 2016;315:801 -10. https://doi.org/10.1001/jama.2016.0287.

[10] Bousselmi H. LES INFECTIONS BACTÉRIENNES CHEZ LE CIRRHOTIQUE: FACTEURS PRONOSTIQUES ET PRISE EN CHARGE [thèse]. Medecine-Tunis; 2020.86p.docx n.d. n.d.

[11] Houissa F, Mouelhi L, Amouri N, Salem M, Bouzaidi S, Debbeche R, et al [Factors predicting mortality in infected hospitalized cirrhotics patients: about 97 cases]. Tunis Med 2012;90:807-11.

[12] Piano S, Bartoletti M, Tonon M, Baldassarre M, Chies G, Romano A, et al. Assessment of Sepsis-3 criteria and quick SOFA in patients with cirrhosis and bacterial infections. Gut 2018;67:1892-9. https://doi.org/10.1136/gutjnl-2017-314324.

[13]Piano S, Singh V, Caraceni P, Maiwall R, Alessandria C, Fernandez J, et al. Epidemiology and Effects of Bacterial Infections in Patients With Cirrhosis Worldwide. Gastroenterology 2019;156:1368-1380.e10. https://doi.org/10.1053/j.gastro.2018.12.005.
[14]Augustinho FC, Zocche TL, Borgonovo A, Maggi DC, Rateke ECM, Matiollo C, et al. Applicability of Sepsis-3 criteria and quick Sequential Organ Failure Assessment in patients with cirrhosis hospitalised for bacterial infections. Liver Int 2019;39:307-15. https://doi.org/10.1111/liv.13980.
[15]Müller M, Schefold JC, Leichtle AB, Srivastava D, Lindner G, Exadaktylos AK, et al. qSOFA score not predictive of in-hospital mortality in emergency patients with decompensated liver cirrhosis. Med Klin Intensivmed Notfmed 2019;114:724-32. https://doi.org/10.1007/s00063-018-0477-z.
[16]Kim JH, Jun BG, Lee M, Lee HA, Kim TS, Heo JW, et al. Reappraisal of sepsis-3 and CLIF-SOFA as predictors of mortality in patients with cirrhosis and infection presenting to the emergency department: A multicenter study. Clin Mol Hepatol 2022;28:540-52. https://doi.org/10.3350/cmh.2021.0169.
[17]European Association for the Study of the Liver. EASL Clinical Practical Guidelines: Management of Alcoholic Liver Disease. Journal of Hepatology 2012;57:399-420. https://doi.org/10.1016/j.jhep.2012.04.004.
[18]Deschênes M, Villeneuve JP. Risk factors for the development of bacterial infections in hospitalized patients with cirrhosis. Am J Gastroenterol 1999;94:2193-7. https://doi.org/10.1111/j.1572-0241.1999.01293.x.
[19]Silvain C, Besson I, Ingrand P, Mannant PR, Fort E, Beauchant M. Prognosis and long-term recurrence of spontaneous bacterial peritonitis in cirrhosis. J Hepatol 1993;19:188-9. https://doi.org/10.1016/s0168-8278(05)80196-5.
[20]Ajayi AO, Adegun PT, Ajayi EA, Raimi HT, Dada SA. Prevalence of spontaneous bacterial peritonitis in liver cirrhosis with ascites. Pan Afr Med J 2013;15. https://doi.org/10.11604/pamj.2013.15.128.2702.
[21]Orman ES, Ghabril M, Chalasani N. Poor Performance Status Is Associated With Increased Mortality in Patients With Cirrhosis. Clinical Gastroenterology and Hepatology 2016;14:1189-1195.e1. https://doi.org/10.1016/j.cgh.2016.03.036.
[22]Weil D, Levesque E, McPhail M, Cavallazzi R, Theocharidou E, Cholongitas E, et al. Prognosis of cirrhotic patients admitted to intensive care unit: a meta-analysis. Ann Intensive Care 2017;7:33. https://doi.org/10.1186/s13613-017-0249-6.
[23]Mackenzie I, Woodhouse J. C-reactive protein concentrations during bacteraemia: a comparison between patients with and without liver dysfunction. Intensive Care Med 2006;32:1344-51. https://doi.org/10.1007/s00134-006-0251-1.
[24]Papp M, Vitalis Z, Altorjay I, Tornai I, Udvardy M, Harsfalvi J, et al. Acute phase proteins in the diagnosis and prediction of cirrhosis associated bacterial infections. Liver Int 2012;32:603-11. https://doi.Org/10.1111/j.1478- 3231.2011.02689.x.
[25]McHutchison JG, Manns MP, Longo DL. Definition and management of anemia in patients infected with hepatitis C virus. Liver Int 2006;26:389-98. https://doi.org/10.1111/j.1478-3231.2006.01228.x .
[26]Singh S, Manrai M, V S P, Kumar D, Srivastava S, Pathak B. Association of liver cirrhosis severity with anemia: does it matter? Ann Gastroenterol 2020;33:272- 6. https://doi.org/10.20524/aog.2020.0478.

[27] Stanley AJ, McGregor IR, Dillon JF, Bouchier IAD, Hayes PC. Neutrophil activation in chronic liver disease: European Journal of Gastroenterology & Hepatology 1996;8:135-8. https://doi.org/10.1097/00042737-199602000-00008.
[28] Angeli P, Wong F, Watson H, Ginès P, CAPPS Investigators. Hyponatremia in cirrhosis: Results of a patient population survey. Hepatology 2006;44:1535-42. https://doi.org/10.1002/hep.21412.
[29] Fasolato S, Angeli P, Dallagnese L, Maresio G, Zola E, Mazza E, et al. Renal failure and bacterial infections in patients with cirrhosis: epidemiology and clinical features. Hepatology 2007;45:223-9. https://doi.org/10.1002/hep.21443 .
[30] Pauwels A, Meunier L, Boivineau G, Martin T, Touze I, Zuberbuhler F, et al. Resistant bacterial infections in cirrhosis: a French observational prospective multicentre nationwide study (RESIST study). Journal of Hepatology 2017;66:S131 - 2. https://doi.org/10.1016/S0168-8278(17)30532-9.
[31] Fernández J, Bert F, Nicolas-Chanoine M-H. The challenges of multi-drug resistance in hepatology. J Hepatol 2016;65:1043-54. https://doi.org/10.1016/j.jhep.2016.08.006.
[32] Rabinovitz M, Prieto M, Gavaler JS, Van Thiel DH. Bacteriuria in patients with cirrhosis. Journal of Hepatology 1992;16:73-6. https://doi.org/10.1016/S0168-8278(05)80097-2.
[33] Navasa M, Rimola A, Rodés J. Bacterial Infections in Liver Disease. Semin Liver Dis 1997;17:323-33. https://doi.org/10.1055/s-2007-1007209.
[34] Société Française D'Anesthésie Et. Probabilistic antibiotic therapy for severe septic states. Annales Françaises d'Anesthésie et de Réanimation 2004;23:1020-6. https://doi.org/10.1016/j.annfar.2004.08.001 .
[35] Fernández J, Gustot T. Management of bacterial infections in cirrhosis. Journal of Hepatology 2012;56:S1 -12. https://doi.org/10.1016/S0168- .8278(12)60002-6
[36] Papp M, Farkas A, Udvardy M, Tornai I. Bacterial infections in cirrhosis. Orvosi Hetilap 2007;148:387-95. https://doi.org/10.1556/oh.2007.27882 .
[37] Runyon BA. Management of adult patients with ascites due to cirrhosis. Hepatology 2004;39:841-56. https://doi.org/10.1002/hep.20066.
[38] Silva M, Laires P, Costa M, Leão R, Roque A, Calinas F. Hospitalization Costs Associated With Liver Cirrhosis. Value Health 2014;17:A365. https://doi.org/10.1016/j.jval.2014.08.812.
[39] Bruns T, Zimmermann HW, Stallmach A. Risk factors and outcome of bacterial infections in cirrhosis. World J Gastroenterol 2014;20:2542-54. https://doi.org/10.3748/wjg.v20.i10.2542.
[40] Schrier RW, Arroyo V, Bernardi M, Epstein M, Henriksen JH, Rodés J. Peripheral arterial vasodilation hypothesis: A proposal for the initiation of renal sodium and water retention in cirrhosis. Hepatology 1988;8:1151-7. https://doi.org/10.1002/hep.1840080532.
[41] Albillos A, Lario M, Álvarez-Mon M. Cirrhosis-associated immune dysfunction: Distinctive features and clinical relevance. Journal of Hepatology 2014;61:1385-96. https://doi.org/10.1016/j.jhep.2014.08.010.
[42] Moreau R, Jalan R, Gines P, Pavesi M, Angeli P, Cordoba J, et al. Acute-on-chronic liver failure is a distinct syndrome that develops in patients with acute decompensation of cirrhosis. Gastroenterology 2013;144:1426-37, 1437.e1-9.

https://doi.org/10.1053/j.gastro.2013.02.042.
[43] Gustot T, Durand F, Lebrec D, Vincent J-L, Moreau R. Severe sepsis in cirrhosis. Hepatology 2009;50:2022-33. https://doi.org/10.1002/hep.23264 .
[44] Arvaniti V, D'Amico G, Fede G, Manousou P, Tsochatzis E, Pleguezuelo M, et al. Infections in patients with cirrhosis increase mortality four-fold and should be used in determining prognosis. Gastroenterology 2010;139:1246-56, 1256.e1-5. https://doi.org/10.1053/j.gastro.2010.06.019.
[45] Kamath PS, Kim WR. The model for end-stage liver disease (MELD). Hepatology 2007;45:797-805. https://doi.org/10.1002/hep.21563.

QUICK SEQUENTIAL ORGAN FAILURE ASSESSMENT IN CIRRHOSIS : INTEREST OF THE SCORE IN INFECTED CIRRHOTICS

Summary

Introduction :

Patients with cirrhosis are at high risk of developing bacterial infections, and the progression is grafted with a number of complications, with an increased risk of mortality. As a result, early identification and prompt management improve survival and are of paramount importance. The qSOFA score has been validated in the general population but is not widely used in infected cirrhotics. The aim of our study was to evaluate this score in this population and its prognostic value as well as its prediction of mortality.

Materials and methods :

We conducted a descriptive, retrospective study including all cirrhotic patients admitted for bacterial infection to the Gastro-Hepato-enterology B department at La Rabta over a period of 5 years. We analysed the bacteriological and evolutionary profile and retrospectively calculated the qSOFA score in order to study the association between this score and mortality during hospitalisation and over a 12-month follow-up.

Results :

A total of 61 patients were enrolled. Our population was predominantly female and the mean age at inclusion was 63±12 years. Viral aetiology (HCV or HBV) was the predominant aetiology (63.9%). Infection was inaugural in 15% of cases. DOA was the main reason for consultation (78.8%). Physical examination revealed ascites, arterial hypotension, polypnoea and an altered general condition in 86.9%, 55.7%, 47.5% and 37.7% of patients, respectively. SIB was present in the majority (80.3%). On admission, the majority of patients were classified as CHILD C (50.8%) and 45.9% had a MELD > 15. UTI (42.6%) and ALI (21.3%) were the most frequent. The infectious agent was identified in 52.5% of patients. BGN represented 81.3% of the germs isolated (*Escherichia coli,* 53.1%). Empirical first-line antibiotic therapy was initiated in 93% of patients, mainly based on monotherapy (88%). Injectable C3Gs were prescribed most frequently (75%). A positive qSOFA (>2) was present in 44% of patients. The median hospital stay was 18 days, with a favourable outcome in 75.4% of cases. One or more complications were observed in 24.6% of patients. Hepatic encephalopathy occurred in 23% of infected cirrhotics, septic DCI (14.8%) and ACLF (9.8%). Forty-one per cent of cirrhotics died during the 12-month follow-up, with an in-hospital mortality rate of 16%. Of those who died, 96% had a qSOFA > 2. A positive qSOFA was significantly associated with the development of septic DCI and ACLF. Similarly, overall mortality was significantly higher in cirrhotic patients with a qSOFA > 2. By analysing the ROC curves of qSOFA score and mortality, the AUROC was 0.953, 0.550, 0.524 and 0.476 for overall, in-hospital, 6-month and 12-month mortality, respectively. prediction of mortality by univariate analysis revealed a significant association with the following parameters: EH, impaired general condition, GCS <15, DOA, CRP and hyponatremia, etc. In the multivariate analysis, the prediction of mortality by univariate analysis revealed a significant association with the following parameters: EH, impaired general condition, GCS <15, DOA, CRP and hyponatremia. In the multivariate analysis, only the development of ACLF and EDC, a GCS<15, and impaired general condition were retained as independent factors predicting mortality.

Conclusion:

This study confirms the seriousness of bacterial infection in cirrhosis in terms of multi-organ failure and mortality. The qSOFA score is a bedside tool for assessing the risk of worsening in these patients. Patients with a positive qSOFA deserve more intensive management and strict monitoring.

Key words: cirrhosis, Score, Mortality, bacterial infections

7 APPENDICES

Tabic 7: International Club of Ascites (ICA-AK1) new definitions for the diagnosis and management of acute kidney injury in patients with cirrhosis.

Subject	Definition
Baseline sCr	A value of sir obtained in the previous three months, when available, can be used as baseline sCr. In patients with more than one value within the previous three months, the value closest to the admission time to the hospital should be used. In patients without a previous sCr value, the sCr on admission should be used as baseline.
Definition of AKI	- Increase in sCr >03 mgi'dl (¿26.5 pmol/L) within 48 h; or, - A percentage macase sCr ¿50% which is known, or presumed, to have occurred within the prior seven days
Staging of AKI	- Stage 1: increase in sCr >0.3 mg/dl (¿26.5 pmol/L) or an increase in sCr >15-fold to 2-fold from baseline; - Stage 2: increase in sCr >2-fold to 3-fold from baseline; - Stage 3: increase of sCr > 3-fold from baseline or sCr >4.0 mgi'dl (353.6 pmol/L) with an acute increase ¿0.3 mgi'dl (¿26.5 pmol/L) or initiation of renal replacement therapy
Progress g of AKI	Progression: Progression of AKI to a higher stage and/or need for RRT Regression: Regression of AKI to a lower stage
Response to treatment	No response: No regression of AKI Partial response: Regression of AKI stage with a reduction of sCr to ¿0.3 mgidl (¿265 pmol/L) above the baseline value Full response: Return of sCr to a value within 0.3 mg/dl (¿26.5 pmol/L) of the baseline value

AKI, acute kidney injury; sCr, serum crean nine; KKI, renal replacement therapy.

Appendix 1: Hepato-renal syndrome in cirrhosis

First name First name : Age: ND:

Sex: M □ / F □

History: COMORBIDITY yes □ - no □ if yes types:

Diabetes □; High blood pressure □; Dyslipidemia □; Coronary □ Heart disease □; Chronic respiratory insufficiency □; Renal insufficiency □

OTHER □ please specify:

Habit: Tobacco yes □; if yes N°: PA - no □

Alcohol yes □ - no □

Etiology of cirrhosis: HVB □ / HVC □ / HAI□ / CBP □ / SD Overlap □ / NASH □ / ethylicü / Idiopathic □ / OTHER □ if yes please specify:

Time to diagnose cirrhosis: months

Functional signs:

Fever □ Chills □ Asthenia□ Abdominal pain□ Diarrhoea □ Vomiting □ Dyspnoea □ Productive cough □

Urinary signs: yes □ no □

if yes: dysuria □ / pollakiuria □/ urinary burning □

Consultation deadlines: days

Clinical signs:

T°: ;- BP: cmHg; - Pulse puls/min; - RF cycle/min;

BMI Kg/m2; - Jaundice □; - General condition: Good □ Fair □ Poor □; Dehydration □ - Ascitesü; Pleurisy □ - OMIÜ; - EH □ if yes stage: Iü / IIÜ ZIIIÜ - Skin lesions □ -

Bronchial rales □
Child_Pugh classification: A □; BП; CП
Score by Meld:
Score q SOFA:
> 2 □
< 2 □
Biology:
CBC: Haemoglobin : g/dl; White blood cells: /mm3
Platelets: /mm3. **CRP:** mg/l; SV mm/h; **blood glucose**: mmol/l **Blood ionogram**: Natremia: mmol/L ;
kalemia: mmol/L; **Uremia**: umol/l; **Creatininaemia**: umol/l.
ASAT: UI/L; ALAT: UI/L; Total bilirubin: umol/l,
Alkaline phosphatase: IU/l; Gamma G T IU/l.
Albumin g/l, TP% INR
Type of infection:
A/ Nosocomial □ Community □
B/ Germ□ if yes
Identified on
Direct examination □ - Culture □ - PCR □ - Biopsies □
PELA □ - Pleural puncture □ - ECBU □ - Coproculture □ - Colic biopsies □ - Puncture of a collection / abscess □ - Blood culture □ - Skin samples□ - Other □ If yes, please specify
Type of germ: Gram-positive □
Gram-negative □
Escherichia coli □ Klebsiella pneumonia□ Enterococcus faecium □ Enterococcus faecalis □ Staphylococcus aureus □ Pseudomonas aeruginosa □ Other Enterobacteriaceae □ Streptococci □ Mycobacterium tuberculosis □ Mycobacterium bovis□ Other □ if yes type:
Antibiogram □ if yes
Sensitive □
Resistant□
Multi-resistan□
C/ TYPE OF INFECTION
1) ILA □
LA study: appearance: citrine yellow □; cloudy □; chylous □; hematic□ Protein : g/l Leukocytes: /mm3 Lymphocytes: %
PNN : % AND PNN/ mm^3
2) Digestive tract infections^
a) **<u>Infectious</u> colitisD, <u>infectious</u> ileitisP** ileocolonoscopy: congestive mucosa □; colonic ulcerations □ Other
b) **<u>Hepatic</u> abscessD - <u>intra-abdominal collection</u>** □ Abdominal CT: location
Size cm; - puncture-drainage □
3) Urinary <u>tract infectionP</u>
4) ECBU: Leukocytes:
/mm3 Lymphocytes: % PNN :
5) Skin infection □

Type: Erysipelas- □, cellulitis- □ si oui siege - phlegmonn if yes siege ; Panaris □; - folliculitis □; Other

6) Pleuro-broncho-pulmonary infection □ if yes

types: ILP □ - Pneumonia - □- Bronchopneumonia □ - Lung abscesses □

7) ENT infection □

Type: Dental abscess □ - Otitis □ - Other □ if yes please specify

8) Other types of infection if yes □ please specify

TREATMENT

I) Antibiotic therapy:

ß-lactam□ if yes: C1G □ - C2G □ - C3G □ - Penicillins □ penicillins with a beta-lactamase inhibitorD Dosage: g/d / Duration : j

Aminoside □ Dosage: g/d / Duration : j

Macrolide□ Dosage : g/d / Duration : j

Metronidazole□ Dosage : g/d / Duration : j

Quinilones Dosage : g/d / Duration : j

Cyclines PPosology : g/d / Duration : j

Other P to be specified Dosage : g/d / Duration : j

II) Puncture □ - DrainageD if yes duration of drainage j.

Length of hospital stay: days

Evolution

Favourable

YES □ if yes:

Disappearance of infectious syndrome □

Disappearance of radiological images □

Negativation of a previously positive bacteriological examination □ Absence of complications □.

NOÜ if no

Encephalopathy □ - Aggravation Of Neurological Signs □ - Occurrence Of Renal Failure □ - Aggravation Of Hepatocellular Failure □ - Hemodynamic Failure □ - Respiratory Distress □ - Other □ specify

Mortality yes □ no □

if yes in hospital yes □ no □

Deadlines: months

Appendix 2: Template

	WHO Performance Index (PS)
0	Normal activity
1	Restretta activity: autonomous and able to do light work during the day
2	Reduced activity of 50%: independent but unable to support a job
3	Confined to bed or a cat more than 50% of the time: reduced autonomy
4	Permanently confined to bed, totally dependent

Appendix 3: WHO score for ¡assessment of general condition

	Y eye response (eye opening)	**Verbal response V**	**M motor response** (to commands, to pain)
1	No	No	No
2	Pain	Sounds	Extension
3	Call	Word	Stereotyped flexion
4	Normal	Confused	Simple bending
5		Normal	Directed to pain
6			Normal

Appendix 4: Glasgow Core Score (GCS)

Assessment qSOFA	score
Low blood pressure (SBP <100 mmHg)	1
High respiratory rate (>22 breaths/min)	1
Altered mentation (GCS <14)	1

Appendix 4: qSOFA score

Paramètres	**Critères**
Fréquence cardiaque	**>90/min**
Fréquence respiratoire	**>20/min ou** **$PaCO_2$ <32 mmHg ou** **nécessité d'une ventilation mécanique**
Température	**>38°C ou** **<36°C**
Leucocytes	**>12 G/l ou** **<4 G/l ou** **déviation gauche >10%**

Appendix 5: SRIS criteria

Score

	Score				
Système	**0**	**1**	**2**	**3**	**4**
Respiration					
PaO2/FiO2, mmHg (kPa)	≥ 400 (53,3)	<400 (53,3)	< 300 (40)	<200 (26,7) avec soutien ventilatoire	<100 (13,3) avec soutien ventilatoire
Coagulation					
Plaquettes, x10³/µl	≥ 150	< 150	<100	< 50	< 20
Foie					
Bilirubine, µmol/l (mg/dl)	<1,2 (20)	1,2-1,9 (20-32)	2,0-5,9 (33-101)	6,0-11,9 (102-204)	>12,0 (204)
Cardiovasculaire	PAM ≥ 70 mmHg	PAM < 70 mmHg	Dopamine < 5 ou dobutamine (toute dose)*	Dopamine 5,1-15 ou adrénaline ≤ 0,1 ou noradrénaline ≤ 0,1*	Dopamine <15 ou adrénaline >0,1 ou noradrénaline >0,1*
Système nerveux central					
Glasgow Coma Scale	15	13-14	10-12	6-9	<6
Rénal					
Créatinine, µmol/l (mg/dl)	<1,2 (110)	1,2-1,9 (110-170)	2,0-3,4 (171-299)	3,5-4,9 (300-400)	>5 (440)
Diurèse, ml/j				<500	<200

Appendix 6: SOFA score

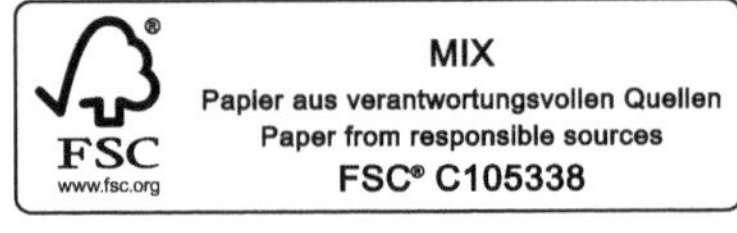

Printed by Books on Demand GmbH, Norderstedt / Germany